ADVANCED CHAKRA HEALING

Cancer

ADVANCED CHAKRA HEALING

The Four Pathways Approach

CANCER

Cyndi Dale

THE CROSSING PRESS
Berkeley | Toronto

THE CROSSING PRESS
A Division of Ten Speed Press
PO Box 7123
Berkeley, California 94707
www.tenspeed.com

Distributed in Australia by Simon and Schuster Australia, in Canada by Ten Speed Press Canada, in New Zealand by Southern Publishers Group, in South Africa by Real Books, and in the United Kingdom and Europe by Airlift Book Company.

Cover and text design by Lisa Buckley Design

Library of Congress Cataloging-in-Publication Data
Dale, Cyndi.
Advanced chakra healing : cancer : the four pathways approach / Cyndi Dale.
p. cm.
ISBN-13: 978-1-58091-170-2
ISBN-10: 1-58091-170-6
1. Cancer—Alternative treatment. 2. Chakras—Health aspects.
I. Title.
RC271.A62D35 2005
616.99'406--dc22
2005021131

Printed in the United States of America
First printing, 2005

1 2 3 4 5 6 7 8 9 10 — 09 08 07 06 05

Contents

Acknowledgments

Can a book be dedicated to its readers? I hope so, because this one is.

I don't see you as a group, rather as individual people who are affected by cancer. Some of you wear faces that I have seen. There's Marlene, who recovered from melanoma to continue raising her four children as a single parent. She used to read comic books every day to cope with the pain of chemotherapy. There's Liu Chen, who took up running after being given a terminal liver cancer diagnosis at age eighty-two. In his words, "I'll go out running, thank you." He lived six more years, dying of pneumonia right after finishing college. To those who have recovered, are recovering, and are living through cancer, I thank you for your strength, for the role modeling that you provide us all.

I think also of those to whom this book is a tribute. There is Ariana, the little eighteen-month-old girl who died of a brain tumor. She died smiling, her last gesture a final touch on her mother's lips, a kiss of comfort to say good-bye. Tony, who passed away at age twenty-one of pancreatic cancer, didn't believe until a few minutes before leaving that he would really die of the disease. Just before passing, he reached for his father's hand and said, "Thank you, Dad, for bringing me into the world." I hold in my heart memories of my friend Ben, who died from bone cancer, still promising to build a healing center for people battling cancer and other diseases. Who is to say he isn't even now attending the world, trying to tell us that the world IS a healing center? I hold precious the memories of my father, happy that his cancer-infested lungs are now breathing the breath of God, not the toxins of disease. I know of these people that cancer couldn't or didn't erase their souls, their spirits. The journey of cancer instead made their real selves clearer. Those who knew and loved them saw through the body, to the light beneath. They gave us all beacons to follow through our own pilgrimage along this state of being called "life."

There are specific people I wish to thank for the preparation and creation of this book, who are also lights in my world. An indescribable thank you to Lily Binns, my editor at Ten Speed, who knew exactly what I needed to write — and rewrite. Lily has made this book, and I mean that. My hat's off to Kristi Hein, who copyedited this book as well as *Advanced Chakra Healing*. Kristi's pointed and poignant comments and perceptive eye caused me many chuckles and a return to the task of rewriting. To Jo Ann Deck, publisher at Ten Speed, and Ellen Sue Stern, my agent and friend, my blessings and gratitude. And how can I thank my friend and pinch editor, Cathy Scofield, who also spent a Sunday afternoon with me over the phone trying to figure out how to best describe the swings of the chakras? Finally, a thank you to my dearest friend, Dr. Robert Qualls, and my son Michael, who both sat in the waiting room at the hospital while my father died. They were playing the board game called "Life," which is a fitting tribute to all who have cancer.

Introduction

I remember when my dad was diagnosed with lung cancer. There were tears in his eyes when he told me. Even though he said, "We'll fight it," I saw only the trembling of his hands. All I could say was, "I'll be with you, Dad." I knew that we were both scared and that neither of us believed in the premise of winning the battle against cancer.

There are thousands of diseases, but perhaps none as frightening as cancer. Cancer destroys. Cancer kills. Cancer is considered all-powerful. Nobody wants to say that they have cancer, because nobody wants to face the seeming death sentence implied by the diagnosis.

Statistics don't offer a great deal of hope for surviving cancer, especially for recovery over time. Statistics, however, aren't personal. They don't describe a child's reaction to her mother's diagnosis, or the empty space left by a deceased loved one. Nor do they illustrate the excitement of a clear blood test or the smiles after a successful surgery. It's time that we pull cancer off the statistical charts. That is why I have developed a new method for healing cancer: the Four Pathways approach, a process for using the ancient and mystical chakra system for accessing four levels of awareness, each a path for self-healing. Through the Four Pathways approach, you can command change. You can produce miracles. You can heal cancer.

I introduced the Four Pathways approach to healing in my guidebook, *Advanced Chakra Healing*. This groundbreaking system is the result of fifteen years of working as an energy healer.

I love my profession. I use chakra knowledge to help people face life problems ranging from relationship confusion to terminal illness. Often, the work leads to life-changing results, even when the person is facing a critical challenge like cancer. A child's tumor might disappear. A runaway teenager might return home to buoy a dying parent. A mother of four children might ease through chemotherapy, still able to tend to her family. I wrote *Advanced Chakra Healing: Cancer* because I know the concepts and practices can and do work to heal cancer or the conditions surrounding cancer.

This book is also, however, a reaction to a lifetime of frustration with the curative methods offered by traditional and even alternative care. We've all noticed that the best of the available medical care doesn't always lead to the best results. This outcome doesn't make sense, given the resilience of the body, mind, and spirit. Our bodies regenerate constantly, so why is it so difficult to encourage extraordinary healing? The simplest thoughts can determine whether we regain health or succumb to disease, so why is it so hard to control our well-being? We are all spiritual beings, so why doesn't this truth ensure physical response?

I found the answer to the latter question amazingly simple. It is this: we don't understand the nature of reality.

The Four Pathways approach calls for a radical shift in looking at reality. It is an approach that does not just request true healing, but insists on it.

To successfully work the Four Pathways approach for healing, you must first transcend the limiting viewpoint of being "the patient." Why curtail your healing by confining yourself to this job description? Patients must patiently wait while other people make them better — or not.

Many of my clients assume that as the developer of the Four Pathways process, I will serve as the pathway healer. They enter my office or open my books and hope that I can make all their problems go away. I can operate as tour guide, instructor, even cheerleader, but not as healer. I can be a friend, listening mate, and healing advisor, but not a miracle maker. Nor will your physician, therapist, or best friend be assigned this script. The Four Pathways process is ultimately an odyssey of self-discovery. When you opened this book, you initiated the process of becoming your own healer. If you stick with the journey of the four pathways, at some point you will emerge as a cancer healer — and perhaps as someone healed of cancer.

Enter the world of the Four Pathways, and you are immediately assigned a new title: that of healer.

This book is organized like a map, a guidebook for the odyssey that cancer invited — or forced — upon you. In Part I, you will be introduced to the ideas and concepts needed to excel at the Four Pathways process and optimize your chances for healing. In Part II, you will learn how to actually travel each of the four pathways of reality, directing and managing energies for incredible healing results.

As you follow the pages in this book, you will find yourself roving highways and byways it's likely you have seldom — or never — seen before. All the terms and ideas in this book were first introduced in the prime reference, *Advanced Chakra Healing* — and the two books are very much complementary companions. I always point out when greater detail is available in *Advanced Chakra Healing*. Know that you can refer to the mother book to apply its concepts to the healing of cancer; in fact, I recommend that you do so for optimum healing. With reference in hand, you can follow the road map within this book to acquaint yourself with the philosophies, ideas, techniques, and attitudes necessary to heal cancer in yourself or a loved one.

I'm excited about this book because I have found cancer to be extremely responsive to pathway modalities. *Cancer* is a universally accepted term for cells that mutate and then eventually overrun the body. The contemporary healing tool kit employs only a few methods to battle this unwieldy giant. Some techniques are effective some of the time. Some cancers are untreatable with any known process. One key reason for such disappointing outcomes is that there are hundreds of types of malignancies, and within these types are indefinite subgroups. Because each person is unique, the type of cancer affecting you or a loved one will also be unique, as will be its causes and effects. No current healing process deals with all the nuances of each individual's cancer.

The Four Pathways method includes the broad range of theories and techniques needed to overwhelm a multidimensional disease like cancer. Cancer is slippery. To really effect a change, you must personalize the healing process. The Four Pathways approach offers the diversity necessary to deal with this deadly and elusive problem. It enhances the effectiveness of all current treatments, including conventional and complementary procedures, while allowing you to also choose from an array of other options. You can therefore tailor a healing program to match your needs, personality, and gifts.

Central to all pathway healing is the idea of working energetically. To heal from cancer, you basically must alter the conditions holding cancer energy in your body, exchange malignant energy for more positive energy, or completely cancel out cancerous energy altogether. To achieve these effects through the Four Pathways approach, you must learn how to read energy. Your tool will be your own intuition, or inner knowing. I will show you how to use your intuition to create pictorial or intuitive energy maps to diagnose or heal your own cancer or the cancerous conditions of a loved one or a patient. This process is called *energy mapping* — a term specific to the Four Pathways process.

One of the main reasons for creating an energy map is to conduct an energetic diagnosis. It's important to define the root origins of a cancer. Knowledge of the source will help you alter the energies that support the cancer; it will become a powerful tool in your healing kit. In the Four Pathways framework, cancer is caused by an energy imbalance on one or several of the pathways. For instance, repressed feelings can inhibit your immune function, leading to conditions that cause or reinforce cancer. An impaired immune system overlooks cancer cells, cancer cells kill off good cells, and the spread of cancer cells furthers immune deficiencies. In this scenario, the initiating cause was an emotional discord, but all sorts of energies can become imbalanced and kick off cancer. If you can pinpoint the energies causing havoc, you can then discern which self-healing options will be effective — or not — for healing the cancer.

Healing energies can come from any pathway. Each of the four pathways operates according to a different set of rules and principles and hosts a plethora of influential and miraculous energies. In this book, I will describe the types of energies composing each pathway so that you can recognize them in your life and use them for healing. Your choices are nearly unlimited, as each of the four pathways is exceptional. On your healing pilgrimage you can draw from energies that are broadly physical, supernatural, magical, or divine.

What are these four pathways? The elemental pathway is primarily physical in orientation. On this level you'll look for concrete causes of cancer and use tangible healing instruments like diet, herbs, and chemotherapy. When based in the power pathway, you'll be playing in the supernatural. Here swirl bright and potent energies forceful enough to produce instant illness — or health. Leap to the imagination pathway, and there you'll greet your magical self, who can create wonders out of wishes. Linger on the divine pathway, and there you'll be greeted with love, the ultimate cure for everything.

How will you journey from pathway to pathway? Through your chakras: energy centers that transcend the three-dimensional world. By the time you are finished with this book, you will have been transformed into a true shift healer, someone able to negotiate chakras so as to visit any world or awareness in the blink of an eye! Searching among four worlds for causes and cures might seem complicated, but think, too, of the expanded choice of remedies you'll have!

No matter which pathway you consult for diagnosing or shift healing (a prime Four Pathways technique), the ultimate goal is the same: to identify the Greater Reality. It is said that all paths lead to the same destination. In the case of the Four Pathways, this is true. All pathways lead to the Greater Reality.

To be truly invested within the Greater Reality, however, you must learn how to recognize your own brilliance. You must accept the fact that healing is a matter of illumination, of lighting yourself from the inside to the outside.

In the Greater Reality, you are already whole. You do not "have cancer," any more than you would be considered "cancerous." You are a special and dazzling being, already healthy and healed.

Cancer invites you into true pilgrimage. Although challenging and hard, the ensuing journey will bring you to all the "stations" or places of self that need love and understanding. As you set about healing yourself, you uncover the needs, powers, and abilities that make you a special human being, a being with a divine mission. In the end, cancer becomes the excuse for realizing your genuine self. In the final analysis, on the Four Pathways cancer is a call to wholeness.

From the perspective of the Greater Reality, it doesn't matter if you are a pauper or prince, young or old, sick or well. You are a vital and important part of the All. You don't need to become "more perfect" to be who you are. Nor do you need to be well versed in math, medicine, science, chakras, energy medicine, or spirituality to work the Four Pathways for healing. You have only to draw upon and believe in yourself. In this endeavor, you are also invited to accept the unlimited help available through the Greater Reality.

The only impediment will be your current mind-set, which, in all likelihood, is framed with doubts and cynicism, the two chief mainstays of Western thinking. "Prove it, and I'll believe it" is a common philosophy. "Cure me first, then I'll believe in the cure" is a corollary maxim. How about trading these negative ideas for ones more true to the soul and the spirit? How about beginning with the thought "I believe in myself" and following with yet another striking idea, "I believe myself"? The power to heal is innate in everyone — including you. Believe in yourself, and believe in what you know to be true. Through the Greater Reality, you can compose a great reality of your choice. You can heal from cancer.

PART *One*

chapter one

Cancer as a Call to Wholeness

"But you look happy, sweetheart. Why would I ask you what's the matter?"
"Just ask me."
He shrugged. "What's the matter?"
She immediately started laughing. "What's the matter? Everything is the matter! Rocks! Trees! Atoms! Even anteaters! Everything is the matter!"

— Dan Brown, *Angels and Demons*[1]

How can anything be good, if you or a loved one has cancer? Nothing matters but the fact of cancer. And yet, the sheer audacity of the disease ushers in a brilliant opportunity. A cancer diagnosis invites us to figure out exactly what does matter.

The Invitation of Cancer

Many people consider cancer to be a one-way ticket to death. In truth, it is an invitation into a new state of being.

When you are challenged by a cancer diagnosis, you can't look to the right or the left. You can't go in reverse. The only way to heal from cancer is to heal through cancer. You must walk forward and deal with what comes next. If you choose wisely, what can come next is entry into a Greater Reality, or paradise itself. Within this Greater Reality, there is no cancer. There is only wholeness. There is healing.

Most religions describe paradise or heaven as a region reached only after death. If you are "perfect" enough, you can enter the heavenly state and dwell in eternal bliss, having passed a certain number of earthly tests as an initiation rite. I would challenge this model for the following reasons. First, paradise isn't a place; it's a state of mind or being that allows the giving and receiving of love. Second, it doesn't exist only on the other side of life; it is actually a frame of knowing that allows for fulfillment and joy in the here and now. It isn't a reward for the afterlife; it is the reality of how you live your life. Third, there are no tests that you must pass to achieve this place or state — you need only accept that you already dwell in the celestial realms to make it so.

Cancer isn't a call to examine the afterlife; it is a directive to look at how you are living your life.

If you or a loved one has cancer, then you know what I mean. Every day becomes precious. Every word counts. Every relationship reflects a kaleidoscope of meaning. Every decision carries weight. Cancer forces an examination of purpose and importance. Cancer reflects the need to live your life as if all of life is a paradise.

The obvious question is this: If this world is heaven, then how can cancer be real? The answer is this: cancer doesn't exist in the Greater Reality. Only love is true in the Greater Reality, and love doesn't allow pain or suffering or cancer. Cancer does exist, however, in the planes of reality that compose the Greater Reality — and these are the forms of reality that we most identify with.

Four levels of awareness or realities combine to create the Greater Reality. I call these levels *pathways*, and each offers a different universal approach to life. Each pathway is unique unto itself and functions according to its own set of rules. Cancer can subsist on each of these four pathways, though its causes and cures differ from one pathway to another.

Although each pathway operates independently, they also intersect. A change made on one pathway forces modifications on all other pathways. This interconnectedness can work to your disadvantage. A disease like cancer can spread from pathway to pathway. But perform a healing on one pathway? The healthy energies can impact you on every level, thus further coaxing you into realizing the Greater Reality.

Healing from cancer requires the ability to shift from one level of reality to another in the search for both the causes of and the solutions for a cancerous condition. Hence I use the term *shift healing* to describe the means for healing through the Four Pathways approach. Through this system, you can stay on a single pathway and support your healing with the modalities and energies available on that level. You can also transport healing energies from one pathway to another and achieve supernatural effects in the here and now. Once you master shift healing, you can then perform the most valuable leap of all — the leap of faith into the Greater Reality, the space of the miraculous.

In this book, you'll be shown how to shift heal. You'll learn how to operate within each of the four pathways of reality, searching for causes of and solutions to cancerous conditions. You'll also become skilled at jumping from pathway to pathway, transferring energies at will. You'll become a master healer; you'll become your own healer.

To instigate your healing, you need to be well acquainted with the instruments in your Four Pathways healing kit. You'll be presented with a set of tools, and later a map, for shifting between realities in order to heal from cancer. These instruments could be called mind-set tools, for they aren't as tangible as surgical apparatus or as concrete as medical devices. Rather, your tools are powers of the mind.

Within each of us are all the abilities and powers needed to heal ourselves. One chief attribute is your intuition, which will show you how to peer into a cancer and understand its causes. If you know what supports a certain cancerous condition, you can determine what actions might support healing. Your intuition is crucial to figuring out healing solutions, as it can predict outcome and effect. It is also the key to energy mapping, in which you'll create pictorial representations of the energies surrounding cancer.

Ultimately, the key to the Four Pathways process is to understand energy. In this framework, as well as in such traditional healing systems as Chinese and ayurvedic medicine, all disease is caused by imbalanced energies. Healing occurs when you move energies into balance. The Four Pathways system provides infinite choices for accessing and directing energies for full healing and, best of all, the means for full initiation into the Greater Reality. From this, the highest vantage point, energies automatically assume their proper order, initiating miraculous effects. In the end, you'll find that all that matters is energy.

A Matter of Energy

Everything in the universe is made of energy. Energy is a combination of two forces: vibration and information. The cells in your fingernails vibrate at a different speed than the cells in your brain. These contrasting frequencies are one indicator of the difference between your fingers and your brain. But all energy also contains data that instructs movement and purpose. As Dr. Paul Pearsall says in his book, *The Heart's Code*, energy is "full of information" that instructs it what to do.[2] Vibration plus information — that is, *informed vibration* — makes up everything in the world.

By itself, energy isn't good or bad. Some energies swirl and form to create a cat; other energies move and play to create a plant. Is a cat good? Is it bad? It all depends on what the cat is doing, doesn't it? You'll call your pet cat "good" when it's quiet and "bad" when it's scratching the furniture. A little bit of a hemlock plant clears up acne; an overdose will kill you.

Looking at health is a matter of deciding which energies are helpful and which are harmful. Just labeling something good or bad isn't going to get you very far. An energy that is "good" on one pathway can be harmful on another pathway. A positive energy in outer space can be dangerous in your body.

To reap the benefits of the Four Pathways system, you must be willing to surrender your old notions of energy and what is good or bad. You must be willing to close your eyes to your judgments against cancer and the beliefs that say it is incurable. You have to believe that something as seemingly concrete and material as a chair or a rose or a tumor is really just a conglomeration of energies, and that — poof! — in the same way that water can convert from liquid to gaseous or to solid and icy form, so can something as frighteningly ugly as cancer transform from one shape to another — say, from something to nothing, from malignant to benign. Shift healing — the art of moving energy from one place to another, or changing it from one state into another one — begins and ends with disrupting the thought that the world is concrete. To create a new reality — say, that which is present in the Greater Reality — you must alter your view of reality.

The Magic of Pathway Thinking

Miracles are not only possible on the pathways; they are also probable. To achieve the magical, you have to see reality differently from what you learned in science lab. You must get outside of the bubble of reality that you see as fixed and immutable if you want to challenge a reality that you don't like.

Growing up, I believed that the only reality was the one that I could touch, hear, taste, see, or smell. When I thought about my home, I envisioned a house on Sherwood Avenue in Edina, Minnesota. I knew my home by the color of the house paint and the toys in the yard.

Now, the idea of home conjures images for me that far exceed the sensory or visual. Home is also a feeling, a sense. I create home with others when I exchange love with them. Just as our conscious awareness of reality or an object in reality expands beyond the physical, so does the entirety of the material world extend farther than the obvious.

Science is now suggesting at least twelve dimensions of reality. Most of these aren't apparent to the physical eye or tactile to your skin. The intangible, however, is always present, even when you're seemingly only engaged in everyday activities. Whether I'm walking through a shopping mall, singing in the shower, or feeding broccoli to my five-year-old son, I am intersecting a few or all spaces in time. While "here," I might also be flying in outer space and reading a book in my past, perhaps even attending my own funeral. The truth is that I live in many times and spaces, in many worlds and realms, simultaneously.

You also live in many worlds simultaneously.

New thinking in science is forcing our brains to bend. We are unlocking our collectively rigid mind-sets to reach beyond the old-fashioned confines of time and space, the thinking that insists that only what you can physically sense is real. Once upon a time we alleged that inanimate objects were immobile and that time flowed in only one direction. We believed in universal slowness, that nothing solid could travel faster than the speed of light, and that a slice of reality once destroyed could never be redeemed.

Now it seems that reality isn't as fixed as this paradigm led us to believe.

What would you say if I told you that the chair you're sitting on is in continual motion? That pieces of this chair, particles of time called electrons, linger as far away as the length of a football field? Maybe even in a different dimension? Did you know that the chair is really only here when you look at it, or that a "non-chair" shadows your seemingly dependable seat? Blink, and your inanimate companion might disappear forever! If some or all of this is true, you might be able to quicken a tumor out of existence, to shift it into a different dimension with the right technique, or to wink cancer out of your body. Scientifically, it's possible.

Spiritually, people have long known about a universal and seemingly invisible reality. The four major world spiritual disciplines — Judaism, Christianity, Islam, and Buddhism — are all based on divine revelation: the psychic revealing of truths from an unknown beyond. For centuries, healers called shamans have summoned spirits from the overworld, the underworld, and unknown worlds to shake diseases off and out of their patients. There are other dimensions, just as there are other worlds and ideas and realities in which dreams really do come true and nightmares are undone.

I remember one of my first encounters with the idea of what is now known as a *nonlinear reality*. I was twenty-one and taking a three-month bike trip in Europe. A few weeks into the trip, I was sorer than I had been in my entire life. My existence had narrowed to a relationship between my bottom and the bike seat, my sense of time was wrapped around meal breaks, and my idea of self as anything but a biker had disappeared with my last long-ago glimpse into a mirror.

One day I was enjoying a much-needed day of relaxation in a little town in Germany. So enamored was I of movement without spokes that I wasn't paying attention to anything but my stretching muscles, when I wandered into a scene that altered my viewpoint of reality for years to come.

An elderly gentleman was centered within a bevy of women and children. He was very stooped. What little hair he had flopped from one side of his head to another, not long enough to even begin to cover his startling blue eyes. In all, his image was macabre and even frightening. He was passing out concoctions from an old sack, the pungent aroma of which I could smell from yards away. I couldn't have imagined swallowing the stuff. Fortunately, consumption didn't seem to be mandatory for treatment. Rather, the mothers were simply wiping the paste on their children, probably in the general vicinity of their maladies. As soon as they were touched by the goop, the children would smile and begin running around. Moving closer, I saw one such swipe of the magic salve make a scabbed-over wound disappear before my eyes. Yet another child, who had been holding her arm in pain, began to toss a ball right after being treated with the remedy. Perhaps the most miraculous result involved a little blonde girl. She had been lying motionless in her mother's arms. I couldn't tell if she was even breathing. Instead of treating her with the remedy, the old man simply held his right hand over her forehead and muttered. The girl's eyes fluttered open. Her pale skin flushed, and she began to twitch. Within a few seconds, she had leaped from her mother's arms and joined the children in play.

There was magic in the medicine. Perhaps the magic came from far beyond the medicine.

Yet another journey found me meeting with one of the last medicine men in Belize. He was well known for his knowledge of jungle plants, especially those that cured cancer. With a group I was leading, we trekked to his home, a small hut in the rainforest.

I was fortunate to be provided a few minutes alone with him for discussion. His eyes were milky with age, but his voice was clear. An American medical doctor was present to translate what he said. What question could I ask? What query was important enough to present? Finally, I asked him how to best work with the medicines for healing purposes.

He paused. I thought that for a brief second the clouds cleared from his eyes, and wisdom shone through. "It is not what you do with the medicine," he suggested. "It is what you allow the medicine to do for you."

Inside out and upside down. In Western culture, we think that the curatives perform the curing. Perhaps healing has very little to do with the substances, tinctures, or bandages used.

Perhaps it's all about the energies that flow between worlds; about the way that we tip truth from one dimension to another; about the connection points between pathways and the Greater Reality.

This sentiment was certainly echoed by an explanation of healing provided me by yet another intelligent elder, this one from the North American Lakota Indian tradition. On a hike with him I paused to hold up a four-leaved plant. "What does this plant heal?" I queried.

Black Oak stopped and reflected. He didn't look me in the eye when he answered, which told me that he was going to share a philosophy rather than a fact.

"Do you not know that there are other places that plants touch than the ones they grow upon?" asked Black Oak. "Sometimes the healing must come from those lands."

It is not what you do with the medicine. It is what you allow the medicine to do for you.

Here again, the same idea: a plant as a connection point between the worlds. An object in which different realms crisscross. I absorbed Black Oak's wisdom, and I wondered if I could learn how to direct the energies between worlds; if I could perceive the worlds between windows.

Yet another healer reinforced for me the idea of reality as a mere construct, the outcome of energies shifting between various planes of existence. This was a brilliant shaman named Malidoma Somé, an author and teacher from Africa. I encourage you to read his books, for he speaks of the reality of other worlds in the rendering of his training as a shaman.

In one of his classes, Somé shared a story involving manhood initiations. As a sign of maturity, the boys in his childhood tribe must be able to tap into the seen and unseen worlds. They prepare for a test of bravery and prowess for dealing with the invisible by spending days, if not weeks, gazing at a tree, until finally they are able to see the Greater Reality beyond the form of the tree. The final test is a task. Each boy must leap physically into the tree, throwing himself into the empty space that lies within all trees. From the outside, the boy would seem to be absorbed into the tree itself; to disappear and, it is hoped, to reappear again.

In relation to his initiation, Somé reported the experience of falling through space, and the challenge of catching onto lines of energy so as not to plummet indefinitely. He passed the test. Some boys did not. Those that did not pass never emerged from the tree.

Westerners could call this experience one of pretend or make-believe. Where, then, do the missing boys go? They go somewhere, and they can do so because they see into a world that a nontribal viewer might not see. Just seeing something as real, however, isn't enough to make it real. These boys see into a reality that is real; therefore they can interact with it in a very real way.

There is a Greater Reality, and the shortest distance to reach it is to follow the path of the Four Pathways.

Why are there four, instead of three or seven pathways? Most cross-cultural healing philosophies speak to the idea of four pathways or directions into Truth. Nearly every culture suggests a foundation for healing based on the four compass directions of north, south, east, and west. In my studies of the Lakota people, the Maya, the Berbers, and certain East Indian and Asian groups, as well as indigenous communities of Siberia, Lapland, Peru, Morocco, Greece, Venezuela, Costa Rica, Belize, Brazil, and the British Isles, I have learned that each of these four directions represents a certain type of energy. You can walk toward the center of a circle from any of these four directions and reach the greater whole.

Spirituality has long seen the limitless possibilities that lie within each of us and has relentlessly insisted on a unified reality. Scientific studies are finally reflecting the potentials that lie within us. Scientifically, we just might be at the point where we can make true this statement by fiction author Kurt Vonnegut: "Science is magic that *works*."[3]

The Science of the Pathways

Imagine that together we are attending a workshop on healing, and the instructor presents these objectives:

- Know the invisible as observable
- Know the concrete as unreal
- Heal by creating dreams that are real

We look at each other in wonderment. "This wasn't what I was taught in science class in school," you observe. I nod in agreement. The teacher watches our reaction, and then smiles.

"I'm not sharing what science has always known," she states. "I'm offering truths that have always been real." She explains that science is finally catching up with spirituality. Pursuits in areas like quantum physics, chaos theory, general physics, the theory of relativity, sacred geometry, and fractal mathematics are substantiating greater truths — the truths that explain miraculous healing and supernatural phenomena. After discussing these matters, our teacher punctuates her point.

I BELIEVE OUR INDIVIDUAL SPIRITS are eternally embraced within a grand being, a force that I call God. This would mean that God — my name for the Divine — is within and outside of me at all times.

The most common analogy is to compare God to love. I can relate to this idea because I am a parent. Would I bring children into this world, only to extinguish them if they don't meet my expectations? Would I destroy a child who is weak or needy? Comparably, would I create a universe only to abandon it? The very fact that I, as a human being, can feel such love for my children, family, friends, and, yes, for the world around me only underscores a belief in immortality.

The thought of a God inside and outside of me marks this God as a midwife, ready to greet me in this world at birth — and to welcome me into another world at death.

Most of us think of the Divine as a universal being, one that is fully conscious and yet endowed with human traits, like the abilities to love, make decisions, and bestow favors. I have faith in a divine being who is very much like this, but I also believe that the universe — that is, the impartial and ordered world around us — is established to carry out the will of the Divine. I believe that this universe is structured for love. This structure can be approached through science, for as mystical as this God is, so too is this God logical.

"In this class — as in the text, *Advanced Chakra Healing: Cancer* — you are being presented with the steps to achieve a singular goal. You are being presented the means to move within reality so as to create a new reality."

Consider the ancient spiritual studies of the Kabbalah, a Jewish mystical practice that links the spirit with the mind. The Kabbalah tells a story of creation that mirrors contemporary theories about the beginning of the universe and also coordinates with advanced mathematical concepts.

The science of tomorrow is the spirituality of yesterday and the math of today.

According to the Kabbalah, creation began when an infinite ray of light entered space, forming ten concentric spheres. These spheres are geometrically and mathematically meaningful, signifying ten basic dimensions. As infinity bends around these spheres, we create a contraction, which in turn creates the "imperfect, finite world within the absolute oneness and perfection of God."[4] Earth is so formed as part of a universe that is in fact a multiverse.

Many scientific ideas embrace these same kabbalistic notions, as do mathematical concepts. One of the Big Bang theories of creation describes an energy that wrapped around a core, pulsing energy, causing an explosion of matter that even now continues to expand. You could say that a "perfect energy" of God birthed the "imperfect energy" that is the universe.

Mathematics joins the story with equations about *sets*. Picture a piece of paper that spreads in all directions infinitely. This is infinity, perfection — "God," if you will. Place a point anywhere on this paper, and you have created a point that operates as a space that is finite. Again, we see a world where the finite exists within infinity.

Ultimately, science and math converge to explain "God." In mathematics there is a concept called the axiom of powers. This axiom states that for each set there exists a collection of sets, which includes all the subsets of the given set. This bigger set is called a power set. Basically, this convoluted concept says that there's always a bigger number than the one that you can think of. You can never attain a place of "largest." There is always a force bigger than the sum of all the forces that we now perceive.

Think of this mathematical law in terms of the power of and possibility for healing.

Our futuristic teacher knows that if you can move inside and outside of time and space you can grasp control of energy. Cancer is about energy. To heal cancer, you have only to change the basics of the energy causing cancer. You need only to work the science of energy to create a magical effect.

You begin the healing process by forgetting your surroundings. That chair? Go ahead and sit on it, but remember that it exists only because you need it right now and for some reason other forces have "decided" that it should exist. Much of that chair's energy is even now dancing around the universe. What if you were to try and sit on the parts of the chair that linger in another realm? What might happen to this chair that you are now sitting on?

There is always an authority that is stronger than the one in charge. There is always a place with energies more potent than those present right now. There is always a cancer treatment superior to those now in use.

You don't have to answer these questions. You only need to let them bend your mind. As your mind stretches and curves, it becomes ready for dreaming. If what is real is only imagined, then what you imagine can become real. Your dreams and desires connect the universe of possibility with the world of the practical. Do you hope for healing from cancer? Can you imagine yourself healthy and whole? Can you dream the dreams that will make it so? Then you are ready for the Four Pathways approach to healing.

The Four Pathways: Doors into a Greater Reality

Energy constantly moves around inside of your body. It is also continuously being changed, rearranged, and exchanged. This fact is the secret to healing. This truth is the reason for miracles. A tumor isn't as solid as you might think. What can be changed can be rearranged; what is solid can be made insubstantial; what is dark can be transformed into light. If you can shift energy at will, then you can shift away a tumor.

Dreaming, hoping, and imagining are, in fact, our most universal healing tools.

It is more challenging than you might think to reshuffle matter. If you were to watch the travels of just one particle of matter — say, an electron — you would wonder at how you might ever comprehend its processes enough to grasp control of even one of its movements. Ed the Electron might blink into your bedroom in one moment, flash into outer space within another second, and then suddenly appear in three places elsewhere simultaneously. It is hard to imagine Ed as sane, much less predictable or manageable.

There is actually a rhythm to what seems random. Ed knows exactly what he is doing and why; at least, the energetic laws guiding Ed are reasonable and rational. You have only to look at reality from a high enough peak to understand the orchestration of all that is — even if the seemingly haphazard event is a cancer condition. With understanding comes the awareness needed to direct energies toward healing.

Complete understanding is possible only at the pinnacle of the Greater Reality. Achieving this level of enlightenment is a goal shared by us all. It's also a lifelong goal and might very well take your entire life to achieve.

So what are you supposed to do right now? How can you work energy for healing in this moment of time? Quite simply, you have only to step back from the Greater Reality and walk the pathways that will get you there anyway.

The Four Pathways I've spoken of are four basic levels of awareness — levels of reality that add up to the Greater Reality. Each pathway is a viable and potent path for healing, and each is accessible to you with the snap of a thought. In fact, there is nothing difficult about working any of these paths, because you already exist upon each of them simultaneously.

The four planes of the Greater Reality are made up of physicality, supernaturalism, creative magic, and divine love. Each pathway functions as its own world, operating according to a singular set of principles and laws. As this book proceeds, I will provide you the tools to enter and understand these differing realms. You will learn how to negotiate healing in each land. Becoming versed in each pathway gives you exponential possibilities for healing. Think of the choices available if you have not just one, but four worlds from which to pull healing energies!

You may dwell on all of these pathways at the same time, but you are probably more acquainted with one plane than with the rest. We each have a natural comfort level with certain ways of seeing reality. Still, you've experienced events on each pathway. Although you can conduct your healing on any of the Four Pathways, it is good to know how to operate in each realm. If stuck, you can then leap to a different plane for assistance.

To help you discern among pathways, I am going to describe a person from each of the Four Pathways. As I do this, imagine yourself as this person. Peruse your past. When have you experienced similar feelings or sensations? When have you also journeyed through time in the same way? How did you react to life's little and big events from these various perspectives? Play along with me, and find out which playgrounds you can most easily play on.

Story One: Jim Bites an Apple

Jim was exhausted. He had been busy at work that day and had skipped lunch. Then onward he went after work, to pick up his daughter at day care and run errands for his wife. Finally, he plunked into a chair at home and started watching television.

By the time he was called to dinner, which his wife had prepared, he was too tired to move. He felt sick to his stomach. When he tried to sit up, his head pounded. "Honey," he said, "I think I've got the flu."

His wife felt his head. "No, you don't have a fever," she said. "What was your day like?" Jim unenthusiastically reviewed the events of the day. At the end of his recitation, his wife smiled. "I have just the cure for your malady," she said, before leaving the room. Puzzled, Jim waited until she returned — with an apple in one hand.

"Here," she said. "You haven't eaten! Your blood sugar is low."

Jim took a big bite of the apple. It tasted good, and he quickly finished it off. Within a few minutes his headache had abated, he was hungry for dinner, and he felt a rush of enthusiasm for the evening.

"As they say, an apple a day," joked Jim.

"Eaten on time, would do even better," his wife added.

Story Two: Reggie Rides a Magic Carpet

He couldn't decide what to be when he grew up. The trouble was, Reggie was now forty years old, and he'd tried it all: carpentry, shoe selling, editing, even dairy farming. Nothing grabbed his fancy, and in due time he would simply quit and drift into yet another profession.

He was at the end of the proverbial rope — not that he wanted to hang himself, exactly, but he didn't see a way out of the endless succession of failures. On a night like all others, he went to bed wondering what he could make of himself; wondering where he would wander next.

This evening proved, however, to be a night unlike all others.

While sleeping, Reggie had the sense of being "pulled out of his body." He looked down at his own sleeping form with marvel and fascination. He'd never realized what he really looked like! Suddenly, he sensed a tug and felt himself being rushed away from the earth. When the speeding stopped, he felt like he was in the clouds. He couldn't see anything, but he felt safe. He couldn't hear anything, yet he sensed the presence of something, someone, with him.

Even afterward, Reggie couldn't explain what happened in this space in between wakefulness and sleep, reality and nonreality. He remembered only that some inner part of him seemed to come to life, and he knew himself as a being with strengths and abilities that far surpassed those he used during the normal day. A vision flashed before his eyes, of himself working in a youth home, helping kids figure out who they really are. Then he was back in his body.

Reggie woke up the next day with joy in his heart. He knew what to do with his life! For a moment he worried about how he was going to find the job that he had imagined, and then he dismissed his cynicism. Something mysterious had transpired during the night. Why couldn't he employ the enchantment of his dreams and create the life he had envisioned?

Indeed, his life did transform. A contact made at an earlier job had connections with a youth home that aligned kids with mentors. After meeting with the head of the home, Reggie was offered the job of running the mentoring program. Magic and meaning came together, mysterious as the process was.

Story Three: Marjorie Undoes the Door

Marjorie was panicked. She had been cleaning her kids' room when they left for school. Eager to finish the job, she had kissed them goodbye without rising from the floor, where she was sorting dirty from clean laundry (a thankless job). Teddy, her oldest, had sauntered off with a final salute, slamming the door behind him.

Now the door was jammed. Somehow, it had been shut at an angle that made it impossible to open.

Marjorie lived in the city, and she had been street-smart enough to put bars on the windows. She now wished that she hadn't been quite so paranoid. There was no phone in the room, no tools for unlocking or unhinging the door, and no other way out. She could only clean for so long.

After a couple of hours, Marjorie felt really stupid — and very frustrated. None of her schemes worked. Then she remembered a television show about supernatural powers. Moms had picked up cars using a hidden, secret strength. Couldn't she do the same?

Marshalling her energies and focusing, Marjorie stared at the door. Then quite simply, she decided that it needed to open. She commanded the door to open. She then quietly walked over to the door and turned the knob. It opened.

Story Four: Susan Stops the Car

Susan was in a rush. She was already five minutes late for a birthday party at her mother's, and she could envision her mother's greeting at the door.

"So nice of you to join us," would be the sarcastic remark. "Could you have slapped more paint on the walls than you did on your clothes?"

Susan had just finished a professional painting job, and had been so enamored of the work that she had forgotten to plan enough time to shower and change. Good thing that she had already picked up the birthday present, which was right — where? She was sure that she had placed it in the car this morning!

Swearing under her breath, Susan veered the car around. She could swing by the corner drug store and find something or other — suddenly, she opened her mouth to

> scream. She had just swung her car right into the path of a large semi truck.
>
> She felt frozen. Even if she had the momentum, there wasn't enough time to avert a head-on crash. All she could do was pray. Almost unconsciously, she began to recite a simple prayer she had learned as a child in Sunday school.
>
> With a scream in mid-air, she suddenly felt a jolt. This is it, she thought. She closed her eyes, waiting for impact, and then — she felt nothing. Opening her eyes, she was startled to find herself, still in her car, on the side of the road. The truck had rushed by without striking her. She knew that she hadn't budged the steering wheel. The truck, now behind her, was speeding away in a straight line. It hadn't braked for her. Something — was it God? — had spared her life. She had been granted a miracle.

Have you ever had the types of experiences depicted in these four stories?

Story One illustrates the first pathway. This pathway runs all things physical. It is the most material of all levels of existence. On it, you search for causes and solutions among the practical, tangible, and concrete. A headache — or a tumor — is caused by matters of matter. It's all about what you eat, do, think, feel, see, and hear. Want to heal? Then get practical! Most of us spend most of our time in this first of the four, the *elemental pathway*. After all, we are made of matter.

Story Two describes the world of creative magic. Reggie experiences a life-changing event — and, yes, even rides a magic carpet — through the influence of his mind's eye on this, the third pathway, called the *imagination pathway*. We've all experienced the touch of the mysterious and inexplicable, the influence of our own imagination. Whether we are creating dreams when we're awake or receiving dream messages when asleep, this pathway broadcasts our innate capacity to create.

In Story Three, Marjorie walks the plane of the supernatural. She begins her morning in typical human fashion, caught up in the humdrum and doldrums of the everyday. An event spurs her onto yet a different pathway, however: one that swirls with the colors, forces, and abilities of the paranormal. Have you too experienced a sudden surge of power? Have you ever seen reality respond inexplicably to your demands and needs — in a way that seemingly breaks the laws of nature? Then you have walked this, the second pathway of power. You have journeyed the *power pathway.*

Finally, we see the intercession of the divine in Story Four, in which Susan is gifted with an unforeseen but much-needed miracle on the *divine pathway*. She is saved, not through any effort of her own, but because of the presence and power of the Divine. Look back in time. Uncover your memory. The Divine, in either a small or a grand way, has served us all. We are all watched over by divine love.

You are already a veteran of each of the Four Pathways. You have been a crusader in the physical world, dynamically interacting with matters material. You have commanded influences far beyond the normal, serving as an instrument of the supernatural. You have flown to the stars in your imagination — probably even plucked a few and brought them to earth — thus experiencing the imagination pathway of creative magic. And like all of us, you have been graced with the miracle of love, provided only through the Divine.

When working with a cancerous condition, it is best to have working knowledge of all four pathways. You might have cancer on one pathway but not on the others. You might find signs of the cancer on two, three, or four pathways. Even if you have cancer on all pathways, you will find that it is rooted in only one of the pathways. It's important to uncover the base cause and pathway of a cancer, if only to figure out which healing methods will be effective. As well, this knowledge provides you the opportunity to move energies from pathway to pathway, thus applying superhuman strength to the practical endeavors you are undertaking for healing.

How might these four different pathways appear? How might they relate to cancer? Take a look.

1. The Elemental Pathway: Physical Reality

The word *elemental* means basic and essential. When you work elementally, you reduce a problem to its minute sources and consider the effects of natural law in diagnosis or in healing. Traditional and holistic science is based on elemental understandings. On this pathway, you might determine the cause of a cancer by considering variables such as pH balance or diet, basic feelings or beliefs, which are covered in chapters 5 and 6, or more esoteric causes like energetic bindings and contracts, which are described in chapter 5. Treatment might include elemental techniques such as surgery, chemotherapy, and radiation; more complementary techniques, like herbal medicine, naturopathy, or color therapies; applications of natural forces such as wind or fire; or the acceptance of healing or guidance from nature beings.

You govern the elemental pathway through *intention*. The harder you intentionally search for a cause, the more likely you'll uncover it. The greater your intention to rid yourself of the disease, for instance, the more forceful your immune system will become and the better your success rate will be.

2. The Power Pathway: Supernatural Strength

This pathway ushers you into the world of seemingly uncanny powers and forces — intense energies that can be directed toward change.

There are many types of forces. Since time began, healers called shamans have summoned spirits, energies from other planets and planes, and even the consciousness of plants and animals to assist them in their endeavors. To use the power pathway, you first need to know what forces exist, so you can determine which might be creating disharmony and which can renew balance.

You then work the power pathway through *commanding.* You are able to move supernatural energies by owning your personal right and power to effect change in the physical universe.

Examples of power pathway treatment include infusing medicines with increased healing powers, releasing inanimate forces that are sustaining a cancer, or calling forth powers and forces that could eliminate the cancer.

3. The Imagination Pathway: Creative Magic

Science is substantiating the existence of an "antiworld" — dimensions, universes, and planes that contain possibilities and choices that don't exist in the third dimension, the one that we believe that we occupy. The connection point between the antiworld and "this world" is the imagination pathway.

The imagination pathway can seem like a dim and mystical land, for it requires making constant decisions about what is real or not. This pathway is best described as the connection point between "this world" and the antiworld.

You connect with this pathway by *imagining.* The intuitive ability to imagine allows you to penetrate the veil that prevents us from seeing into other worlds. Through the perception of the imagination, you can release what you don't like in this world and exchange it for what you want from another world. The sudden disappearance and appearance of latent possibilities create the imagination pathway's magical quality.

In many ways, the imagination pathway is the most personally miraculous of the four. The power of faith is made clear when you translate cancer out of your body and exchange it for healthy cells. You rely solely on your own gifts to operate on the imagination pathway, but how strong they are!

4. The Divine Pathway: Awakening to Love

The divine pathway presents itself as a still, yet ever-moving space in which only love is real. Here you heal cancer when you free yourself from lies and illuminate truth.

Life presents us all with seven basic lies, which we must each confront in order to recognize, embrace, and heal through divine love. These lies are universal in nature, involving the presence and adverse affects of evil, death, judgment, misused power, suffering, false miracles, and endings. Once you understand that these lies — such as a belief in evil or death — are mere illusions, truth floods you with tangible and living spiritual energies that meet the need underneath the cancer. Cancer is simply a question mark, an arrow pointing at a place within that doesn't understand the nature of divine love.

On this pathway, you activate healing through *petitioning.* Petitioning isn't the same as begging. Petitioning involves asking for that which you know as your birthright. You receive healing because it has been promised. The divine pathway is the place of miracles, the space of knowing. It is the reality that science cannot completely explain, because it is from here that the basis of all science flows.

Chakra Shifting through the Pathways

When seeking to heal from cancer, you can work just one, a few, or all of the pathways. You can remain on any one of the four levels permanently or for a time period, or you can shift among them at will. *Shift healing* is the term I use to describe the movement of consciousness or energies between pathways.

After you learn about the pathways, it's relatively easy to shift among them. The four pathways are connected like a multidimensional chessboard. You don't need antigravity boots to swing from level to level; you need only to use your chakras.

Chakras serve as portals between the Four Pathways. *Chakra* is an ancient Sanskrit word that means "spinning wheel of light." Indeed, if you could examine a chakra with your naked eye, you would see a whirling tornado of multicolored energies. Most of us cannot distinguish chakras or energy with our physical eyes, however, and so we must learn to rely on a deeper sense of perception when energy healing. We must employ our innate psychic powers to observe the innermost workings of reality. These abilities enable us to see, sense, or hear information that enables us to serve as an energy healer. As perceived physically, each of the twelve basic chakras, seven of which are located directly in the body, will appear as a distinct color, as the energies contained within or used by each operate at diverse frequencies.

Although chakras all share the same structure, they have unique functions. Each chakra governs a different set of bodily, mental, emotional, and spiritual functions and can therefore be accessed to make changes in any part of your life.

Chakras boast a vital role in pathway healing. They connect all the pathways. Not only do chakras emanate from and around your body, but they also run frequencies that can transfer through all dimensions. If you can "enter" a chakra through your intuition, you can direct your consciousness from pathway to pathway and move energy from place to place.

The easiest way to grasp what I mean is to return to your picture of our multidimensional chess game. Look at this game in 3-D. Each pathway is a board. All four boards are stacked atop each other but are interconnected by an "elevator shaft" called the energy system, the key set of organs within this system being the chakras. You can travel through your energy system to any pathway at will simply by shifting your mind-set, but the easiest tools to use are your chakras, namely because the chakras are able to change energy from one speed or form to another — a vital ability in pathway healing.

Chakras convert fast energy to slow energy. Fast energy is vibrating information that travels faster than the speed of light. It is also called psychic energy. In quantum physics, the basic packet of psychic energy is the tachyon. Slow energy is vibrating information that travels slower than the speed of light. It is also called sensory energy. In quantum physics terms, the core unit of sensory energy is the quark. All chakras are able to receive, interpret, send, and sometimes even transform psychic energy or tachyons (fast energy) into sensory energy or quarks (slow energy) and back again. This means that through your chakras you can make energy appear or disappear. Conceivably, you could "poof away" a tumor or materialize healthy immune cells. By programming your chakras energetically, you can attract universal energies supportive of healing, or eliminate bodily energies that are harmful to your health. By peering into your chakras, you can diagnose an illness or pinpoint the exact cause of it. By moving energy through your chakras, you can direct energy so as to ensure a positive outcome.

To perform shift healing, you'll be learning about several subjects. Anyone can learn how to move energy into, out of, and through their chakras, because everyone is intuitive. Intuition is the ability to consciously manage the flow of psychic or sensory energy. You'll be taught how to access and apply your personal intuitive gifts in chapter 5, thereby preparing you for pathway healing. You will also study very specific terms and techniques for conducting chakra changes throughout this book. To deliver healing through your chakras, you will gain knowledge of various ways to manipulate energy through them.

The primary means for energy healing through the chakras entails working with chakra motion, speed, spin, form, and charge. A healthy chakra moves at a particular speed, in a certain form, with a specific spin, and in a decided motion, all of which enables it to get its job done. You can often determine the source of an illness, including a cancerous condition, by evaluating your chakras for problems. A chakra that is off-spin, for instance, might be holding some of the energies causing the cancer. If you can figure out what might make the chakra spin correctly, you can potentially make progress in healing the cancer.

Cancer is held in one of three main types of energy charges. The basic units of physical matter are electrons, protons, and neutrons. These three core energies hold different charges, respectively negative, positive, and neutral. You will come to see that all cancers boil down to an "off" or imbalanced charge, or to harmful information held within charged particles. Diagnosing the charge of a cancer is a useful tool in figuring out healing techniques.

You will learn many ways of evaluating a chakra for its health and well-being. Some of these methods will involve the use of your intuition to check for chakra tones, colors, symbols, numbers, and other indications of health or illness. Shamans and metaphysical healers have employed these concepts since the beginning of time. They work. Why not make them work for you?

Chakra techniques will obviously work in the chakras, but they are also applicable for healing through the various other energy bodies in the energy system. Your energy system expands throughout all four pathways, but the organs available can differ from pathway to pathway. In general, you have a lot of energy bodies on the elemental pathway, only a few on the power pathway, almost none on the imagination pathway, and several on the divine pathway. The exact number, type, and function of energy bodies available on each pathway differ because different types of energies are available on each plane. On earth, for instance, you need eyes to see and ears to hear. If you shift to a planet made of only tones, you won't need eyes — only ears.

There are only two major energy bodies that cut through all four pathways: the chakras and the auric field. In general, chakras regulate your "inside self," while your auric fields run your "outside self." Similar to the chakras, each layer of the auric field regulates a different type of concern. To perform its special function, each layer of the auric field or auric band, as they are sometimes called, runs at a particular frequency. Your auric field in its entirety comprises twelve bands of various frequencies, which begin in your skin and emanate way beyond your physical body.

Like the chakras, your auric fields operate in all four pathways. They perform the same generic function in each pathway: to provide protection and boundaries, and to attract energies required for health and happiness in support of your earthbound, spiritual mission. These auric fields will look slightly unique in each of the pathways, as they will be working with energies special to that pathway.

Pathway healing will frequently call for working with your aura in tandem with your chakras, because each chakra is paired with a fellow auric band. While your chakra is busily attending to business at home (that is, in your body), its partnering field is taking care of the world at large. For instance, one of your chakras might be boosting your immune system to better fight cancer cells; its sister auric band will support the cause by transforming waste products into tachyon particles, thus clearing your body of debris.

Working via your energy bodies is an exciting and dynamic process. I have found no other healing method to be as effective, quick, or enjoyable. When chakra-based healing is coupled with pathway shifts, watch out! From the stance of our everyday life, a tumor can appear to be a giant, unmovable boulder. From a higher lookout point, that tumor is a small dot, easily erased if addressed correctly. A breath of truth from one pathway can seem a mighty gale in another pathway. Shifting through the chakras is equivalent to reducing a lake full of water into a cup, so as to more easily move it. The outcome? Often miraculous.

chapter two

Locating Cancer within a Greater Reality

I contemplate the vastness, behold the black sea, the darkness, the cold and the lights. . . . Yet the sun shines.[1]

— Dean Koontz, *By the Light of the Moon*

If cancer has touched you, then you know how easy it is to let it take over your life. Almost everything about cancer seems overwhelming. Coping with it can be a staggering endeavor, as it seems to twist and shape every aspect of reality. In this chapter, we'll look at the reality of cancer, including the way it has seemingly invaded the human world — and your life. We'll also look at the nature of a Greater Reality, one in which cancer is more similar to a breeze than a wind, a sentence rather than a book, an invitation versus a eulogy. We'll look to the proverbial "silver lining in the clouds," the place where the sun always shines.

Cancer: A Shift into Wholeness

Are you a man? Stand next to another man. One of the two of you will get invasive cancer during your lifetime.

Are you a woman? Picture yourself having coffee with two woman friends. One of the three of you will get cancer sometime in your lifetime.

Lung cancer is the most prevalent killer, with breast cancer second for women and prostate cancer for men. Add colon and rectal cancer to this list and you have what's called "The Big Four" — the major killer cancers. These and other types of cancers have become a major cause of death in the modern world. In fact, cancer has now surpassed heart disease as the leading cause of death in America among people under age eighty-five. It's something that we will all face during our lifetime, if not personally, then through a loved one.

One of the most gripping facts about cancer is that statistically, it's a hard disease to cure. Although the death rate from cancer has technically decreased slightly over time, the only major stride in cancer recovery has occurred among childhood cancers. Measured accurately, the percentage of Americans dying from cancer is about the same in recent years as it was in 1950 and in 1970, despite a $200 billion War on Cancer campaign conducted since 1971.[2] These government and private monies haven't fazed cancer. The annual death toll from cancer in America has risen 73 percent in a half-century — over one and a half times as fast as the increase in the American population — even though death rates for conditions such as heart disease and stroke have been slashed 59 percent and 69 percent, respectively.

In fact, the age-adjusted annual rate of cancer death has increased 8.7 percent in recent decades. Despite decades of intense research on improving treatment of cancer, once a cancer has spread, "chances of survival are scarcely better than they were three decades ago."[3]

Given these odds and the challenges faced by medical science in curing cancer, how would you respond if I told you that the secrets in this book could "cure" your cancer? That the mysteries of energy mapping, the process described in this book, can provide you the means for making this deadly disease disappear for you personally?

I've seen it happen. I've witnessed individuals who had been given a death sentence "rising up and walking," cancer free. I've received calls from clients with whom I've worked over the phone, reporting the disappearance of a cancer untreated by any other method than the ones described in this book. I've connected with clients who continue to be affected by cancer, but now live pain free or free from the fear of dying, able to live the rest of their lives in peace. And I've walked some clients through the hallways of life into death, their last months full of meaning and purpose. Though this part of life's journey is done alone, Divine Love ensures a companionship hard to understand by those of us caught up in the details of life.

I can't predict exactly how the revolutionary concepts and techniques in this book will work for you, but I can assure you of the truth of these two statements:

- Current cancer treatments aren't winning the war against cancer. There's no single known and accessible cure or treatment that works with surety for all people.
- Cancer is a reality. If you want to change the reality of cancer, you must change the reality that created the cancer. Using the ideas and techniques of the Four Pathways approach to healing, you can shift your reality — and possibly your cancer — out of physical existence.

Isn't it worth a try?

You are worth the time and energy necessary to learn how to be your own healer. It might not be easy. It's taken a lot of energy to create or substantiate the reality that you live within right now. Think of what might happen, however, if you were to apply a small amount of the energy going into sustaining your current life reality — one that includes cancer — into the creation of a new reality — one that doesn't embrace cancer. How about wellness instead of malignancy?

The core method for achieving this result through the Four Pathways process is shift healing. Shift healing isn't hard. You change realities all the time. To shift means to exchange one idea, reality, or concept for another. Have you ever ordered a meal at a restaurant and had the waiter substitute a baked potato for french fries? Then you have shifted reality; you have exchanged something that you don't want for something that you do want.

Do you really want cancer? If not, know this: there are ways to shift or exchange cancer, or a life with cancer, for health and a life of joy. At this time in your life, cancer may be a part of your reality, but there are lots of different ways to experience, know, live with, and even heal it.

Cancer may be a reality, but it doesn't have to be one that you live with — or one you necessarily have to die from.

Cancer: A Choice between Realities

You are not your cancer.

Cancer reflects a deeper need, one that points to a wholeness of the self waiting to be realized. Meet this need through means other than cancer, and the cancer doesn't need to be there. This is one of the philosophies of the Four Pathways approach to healing.

How can cancer meet a need? Years before I understood the concepts explored in this book, I worked with a woman with uterine cancer. Diana had six sons and a loving husband, and no woman friends. She had tested positive for uterine cancer the previous year.

When Diana entered my office, I instantly liked her. She was a tall, healthy-looking blonde, with a quick and deep laugh. For all intents and purposes, Diana didn't look like a poster child for cancer. She was so vibrant, it was hard to imagine her reality: the mornings spent throwing up in the toilet after chemotherapy, the tears shed as her hair fell off onto the floor. I wanted to help Diana get better. I thought it might be a relatively easy process, for Diana said that she wanted to get better.

During our first session, I probed for issues that might underlie Diana's cancerous condition. A few minutes into the discussion, I thought, *Aha!* Diana had contracted cancer a month after her mother had died. I intuitively sensed that these two situations were related. Diana did, too.

As soon as we began talking about her mother, Diana broke down and cried. "I want to join my mother," she sobbed. "I've never felt like anyone has loved me as much as she did."

Diana had an almost overwhelming love for her mother, who had been the only woman in her life with whom she had really bonded. Even throughout childhood, Diana had preferred male companionship to feminine friendships. Some twist of fate had gifted her with only male children, and even though Diana desperately cared about her husband, sons, and male friends, it was her mother who made her feel whole and loved.

Energy diagnosis is often a matter of putting puzzle pieces together. Diana's mother had died; psychologically, Diana longed to be with her mother. It was impossible for her mother to return to life. That left only one choice: for Diana to join her mother through death. Another clue to Diana's deeper concerns was the location of her cancer. Cancer often strikes the part of the body that holds or reflects the causal issue. Where are women most bonded, especially as mother and daughter, but through the womb? For Diana, the sac that gave birth was now a potential exit portal for death.

I explained to Diana that perhaps, deep in her subconscious, she had decided to die in order to get her mother's love. Diana affirmed my suggestion. When directly asked if she would rather live and make peace with her mother's death or die in order to reconnect with her mother, Diana affirmed death — even though she had originally stated that she wanted to get well.

She passed away within three weeks.

I didn't know then what I know now. As do most of us, I was only operating on one level of reality. Though I offered Diana a perspective that provided esoteric and psychological understanding, the wisdom didn't alter her subconscious decision about dying rather than living. To help her, I would have had to assess Diana on other planes — or pathways, as I call them — of reality and find a solution elsewhere.

Whenever someone who has cancer enters my office, I remember Diana. I pay homage to Diana, because my brief time knowing her taught me much. She showed me that there could be valid internal reasons for contracting and even dying of cancer. Her situation forced me into humility. Even with the best of motives and intentions, I could not make Diana change her mind. For her, cancer was a doorway into meeting a deeply important need. She showed me that I'm not in charge of healing another person; that no "healer" can heal another being.

Her death also forced me to examine my worldview and skill base to uncover what else I needed to learn. Without meaning to, I had let Diana down. Although I had joined her "where she was at," within her current reality, I had not invited her to examine her "other selves" — aspects of Diana that might exist on other planes. Perhaps, equipped with understandings and energies from one of the other pathways, Diana might have come to understand truths that could have altered her subconscious choice of death. What might have happened if she had merged onto the power pathway, even met her mother's spirit there, so as to command forces for change? If she had peered into another reality on the imagination pathway, finding a purpose for her life path? What if I could have facilitated a true meeting of her and her mother's spirit through the divine pathway, the place of oneness among all?

I know that cancer is often, if not usually, caused by horrible turns of fate. It all too frequently strikes people who have no desire for the disease at any level of their being, such as very young children. Such situations call for even more tenacity in finding assistance throughout the pathways. When the cause of a cancer is outside of the self, of necessity you must engineer energies from external as well as internal sources for healing.

No matter the reason for a cancer, however, I now know that inside every cancer victim is a Diana. Inside each of us is a person who is crying out for help and, ultimately, love; who is requesting to be seen for who he or she really is; who is hoping that cancer can be transformed from something causing tragedy to an invitation into the profound. My experience with Diana also showed me that my true job really involves only one task: to reveal the truth that cancer is a call to recognizing the wholeness that already exists within each of us.

The Continuum of Cancer

One key to healing from cancer is remembering that cancer is not the beginning, nor is it the end, of who you really are. Cancer is a condition. A condition is a mode of existence, one usually characterized by hardship. Cancer causes all kinds of hardship, including physical pain and discomfort, emotional trauma and grief, mental strain and confusion, and spiritual questioning and doubt. Yet you existed before your body created cancer, just as you will continue to exist beyond the condition of cancer and the adversity that it causes.

It's common for people with cancer to suddenly feel like they have been transformed, overnight, from a healthy person to an unhealthy person. We ought not to give cancer that much power. None of us is ever totally healthy, from a purely physical point of view. At any given time, our bodies are infested with germs, dangerous organisms, dead cells, waste products, and, yes, cancer cells. We are always "unhealthy" or "imperfect," if truth be told. At the same time, we are also continually healthy. The body is maintained by the proper exchange of salts, sugars, proteins, fats, and water. It is strengthened by nutrients and our own positive attitudes. It is nourished by our dreams and spiritual beliefs. The condition of cancer is only one process within a sea of other processes that mix and swirl within us.

Of course, cancer is a very loud process. Whereas many other physical routines simply sigh, cancer shouts. And this is good! If you or a loved one has contracted a cancerous condition, you must listen! What is the cancer trying to say? What need is it pointing to? What need is the cancer meeting? What is another way to meet this perceived need?

I'm sometimes asked how contracting a physically based disease such as cancer can be meeting a need. In purely concrete terms, consider one of the main causes of cancer: carcinogenic properties. The body requires sustenance; cells die unless they are able to absorb and utilize the nutrients, oxygen, and other elements provided them. Toxic poisoning by intense radiation, long-term smoking, or chemical exposure erases the cells' ability to process these nurturing elements. Lacking nutrition, cells die — or mutate. Cancer cells are mutated cells.

The presence of cancer is a cry for nourishment, a basic need that has stopped through the interference of poisons. Cancer isn't the initial cause of the need. It's a result of a need going unmet.

In the case of toxicity, the need might be physical, but the cure for physical illnesses isn't always available or workable through physical means. Very few people survive severe radiation poisoning.

Although cancer might be caused physically (as well as through other means), the physical cures we're now using aren't reliable. We might as well give up on the search for a cure for cancer, except for one fact: we coexist on several levels of reality all at once. This means that you aren't limited in protocol to the treatments available in a doctor's office. We aren't confined to the ideas of only the three-dimensional reality. We are free agents in this place called the universe. We are citizens of a much greater reality.

If cancer is choking off your life energy, killing your healthy cells, or stopping you from breathing, you need to feed the parts of yourself that can reenergize your life energy, strengthen your healthy cells, and reinvigorate your lungs. If you believe that you are limited to your body, you may be missing out on many healing opportunities. You won't be able to reach beyond the boundaries of the body or plunge deeper than the diagnosis of death for assistance. You'll find it hard to muster the strength to search for spirit or access emotional powers. *If you don't notice that you are not your cancer, you might allow yourself to become your cancer.*

You can be ill and considered whole simultaneously. As I've already stated, so-called "healthy people" already are! No one questions the health or wellness of someone who shows up at the health club to play tennis, even though he or she harbors millions of germs. An amputee is legally and morally considered a whole person, even if he or she no longer has a particular body part. By accepting your innate wholeness, you actually call more health into being.

By knowing that you exist on planes beyond the physical, you open the doors to the powers and forces of other places. By understanding that you already exist on multiple levels of existence, you invite the awareness of these "other selves." These wiser, more powerful selves might make the difference between dying and living, or dying unhappily versus living completely. Truly, by accepting the self who is whole within the Greater Reality, you welcome more wholeness into the here and now. You allow the matter of energy to create the magic of healing.

What's the Matter with Cancer? (Answer: the Matter of Cancer)

As I've explained, from a Four Pathways perspective, cancer is energy. A cancerous tumor only seems substantial because we are used to seeing it as solid and concrete. There is actually more empty space in a cancer tumor than there is mundane matter. Even then, you can see only a tiny portion of this cancerous matter under a microscope. Most of the matter of cancer isn't very material at all.

To heal cancer through the Four Pathways approach, it is valuable to better understand the basics of matter. Matter is a composite of vibration and information; hence the term we introduced in chapter 1: *informed vibration.*

What exactly are the units of matter that hold the messages that tell one cell to be a useful liver cell, and another to transform into a destructive cancer cell? To answer this question, we're going to enter the relatively new world of quantum physics — the most useful model for explaining how to conduct Four Pathways healing.

The term *quantum physics* originated with the discovery that although there are many types of energies, all of which come in a variety of sizes, they are all composed of particles. Particles are tiny bits of energy. There are larger particles called molecules and parts of molecules called atoms. There are also subatomic particles. Scientists currently guess there are thirty-two types of these minute particles called quanta. In a few more years, we'll probably discover dozens, if not hundreds more. Studying quanta is the basis of a relatively new brand of physics called *quantum theory*; the ideas it articulates are the foundation of this book.

Some quanta move faster than the speed of light; others move slower. Some can even freeze and allow time to flow around them. Think of what you could accomplish if you could change the speed of information. You could pulse a cancer cell out of existence before it is created. You could freeze it forever so it cannot spread. You could slow it down until a traditional cure could be found.

We used to think that matter was trapped in time and space; that it couldn't go faster than light, nor could it escape the clutches of linear time. But this idea was recently disproved when scientists at the NEC Research Institute in Princeton, New Jersey, caused a pulse of light — a collection of waves — to travel so fast that it escaped the test chamber before entering![4] Recent research is also establishing the potential of bringing light to zero point, or standstill. By "freezing light," several researchers showed that you can store light and its energy for a brief time.[5]

There are many fast- and slow-moving quanta. One fast-moving type is the tachyon. In the third dimension, the world of form that we physically occupy, tachyons move energy psychically. Psychic energy is merely information that travels faster than the speed of light and, because of this, breaks the spacetime laws. Applying psychic energy correctly, you could predict the development of cancer and even wish away a tumor before it establishes itself. We use intuition to work the Four Pathways because it is a way to harness the speed and knowledge of the psychic dimensions. By controlling the tachyons that create cancer or those that could shift it away, you can magically manage your healing process.

Although tachyons are so fast as to appear still, quarks are one of the many quanta that progress at a relative snail's pace. Quarks move slower than the speed of light and support sensory energy — the stuff of conversation, sight, and movement. The same information might be contained within a tachyon or a quark, but speed creates the difference in perception.

Logic says that if you want to make a tumor disappear quickly, you work with tachyons instead of quarks. Then again, the quarks and the tachyons connected to cancer might be programmed with very different information. You must change the data in both worlds if you're going to alter a cancerous condition.

Particles are dots of energy; their kissing kin, waves, are flowing streams of energy. Both particles and waves move information across great distances. Particles can jump from one dimension or plane to another, or shift from fast to slow gear. Waves move information long distances and across vast spaces. In general, waves can make big changes rather quickly, simply because of their immense strength; particles must pick away at a problem.

Energy can talk to other energies and actually change their forms and functions. For instance, a particle can interact with another particle and, based on the ensuing discussion, suddenly decide to turn into a wave. A wave might be dillydallying in space, collide with a particle, and be so shocked that it becomes a particle. A wave might be sweeping through your house, carrying multiple particles that you can't see. Then you think a certain thought, and a particle separates from the wave, suddenly "proving" your thought as accurate. Or maybe two waves blend into a completely new wave that has an entirely different function than either had independently. All of these energetic configurations — and the infinite number of others that are possible — can be achieved through the Four Pathways approach. The core idea to understand is that of vibration. Working vibrationally is the key to

By understanding that you are more than your body, you encourage outreach into the different parts of yourself, which can in turn add their powers to bolster your healing. You might learn how to focus your emotions and strengthen your resolve as you undergo chemotherapy. You could exchange a negative belief for a positive one and thus enhance the effectiveness of your immune system. You might follow the message in a dream, which could direct you toward the treatment best for your body. You might figure out that an already-healed self exists aside of you and simply decide to become that self. Or you might wake up one day, notice that the Divine has been holding your hand your entire life, and allow in the love that has always been yours to receive.

controlling particles or waves, the core packages of the information that can both cause and heal cancer.

The Vibration of Cancer

Vibration is movement that occurs with direction. Sound waves are certainly one form of vibrating energy, but so are radio waves, light, and any other type of oscillating energy.

Everything in the universe vibrates. A vibrating object's rate of intensity can be determined by the information encoded within it. Therefore, you can change the vibration of an energy and thus alter its information. This means that healing cancer can involve changing vibration or information.

Most of us think of vibration as orderly and uniform. When you pluck a violin string, you are most aware of the sidewise movement of the string. Depending on the thickness and length of the string and the intensity or velocity of the plucking motion, you will hear a certain tone. This tone is produced by the information of the string vibrating through time and space. To the naked eye, the string is only moving back and forth, but it's actually moving in several directions. In fact, each particle in the string is spinning. Most particles are spinning the same way and in the same geometrical pattern, but some will be moving in opposing or creative oscillations.

The "unified" vibration of a moving particle, wave, or other unit of energy is called a *frequency*. Orchestras tune to the frequency of the note A. When the violins, violas, cellos, and other instruments are tuned to the same frequency, they play melodically, and we're happy to listen. Organs in your body also are attuned to an optimum frequency, as are your cells, your soul, and your mind. If an organ is playing out of tune with the rest of the body, we call the result a disease — a "lack of ease" within the system. When a cell is really out of tune, when it can't even run a single frequency, it's called a cancerous cell.

If removed from the body, a cancer cell isn't a particularly lethal energy. Unless it's supported by other energies, it will simply die. Dangerous cancer cells are those containing information that makes the cell vibrate at a frequency that disturbs the body's normal function. I believe that killer cancer cells are those that don't even vibrate at a modulated or single frequency; instead, they are erratic and frenzied. The more powerful these out-of-tune cancer cells and the greater they are in number, the more effect they have. Ever hear what happens when the only violin in a pit orchestra is out of tune? The entire ensemble sounds wretched. If an entire section of violins were off, you'd leave for home!

Did you know that you run on your own *harmonic*, a set of undertones and overtones that emanate from your inner self? Your inner self, also called your spirit, runs on a frequency based on a spiritual truth. When this truth regulates your entire self, you are happy and healthy. Within your harmonic are several tones or subfrequencies. These must all be tuned to your core frequency to prevent imbalance. Any part of you in discord with the core harmonic is vulnerable to disease. Cancer results when certain cells go out of tune with the rest of your body and ultimately with your spiritual self.

Disease always involves inaccurate information, but it also involves destructive vibrations. We are all exposed to a variety of vibrations; some are health inducing, and some are not. All healing involves using vibration along with information to establish a pattern for health.

Through the pathways, we learn to isolate the threatening vibrations and emphasize the healthy ones. When working the elemental and power pathways, we get very particular about frequencies and vibrations. These pathways are a lot more detailed. We have to assess each and every vibration for accuracy. On the imagination and divine pathways, you can work more generally and simply direct all frequencies and vibrations to match the personal harmonic.

Other Energy Factors in Healing

There are several other factors to consider when working the pathways to heal cancer with particle and wave theory.

Time and Space Many scientists now believe that there are at least twelve dimensions, interconnected by "strings." This means that one part of you might exist in the first dimension and be linked to another part of yourself in, say, the sixth dimension, through either a "quantum string," a tiny particle, or another reality. Your body dwells largely in the third dimension, and if you could conceivably pull the right strings, you could flush a part of a cancerous tumor out of your body and into another dimension or the antiworld.

Comprehending this idea depends on seeing time and space differently. According to a theory called loop quantum space, space forms points and lines called *spin networks.* Because these points and lines keep moving around, scientists suggest that the geometry or form of space is constantly shifting. Time is like a series of tick-tocks in a clock, but the tick might occur in one dimension at noon and the tock in another dimension in the next second. Time doesn't exist between the tick and the tock.[6]

If time isn't consistent, then you can potentially alter the past, present, or future. You could change the conditions that formed a cancer tumor so you don't have it anymore. If space is discontinuous, you could move an object from one space to another. Wouldn't you rather that a child's paper doll have cancer, rather than the child itself? Working on the Four Pathways lifts you out of the standard third-dimension ways to heal cancer by allowing you to shift time and space.

Fields and Forces Everything is in motion, and motion produces a field around all objects, animate or not. *Fields* are energetic extensions or waves that emanate from their source. Some fields create *forces,* such as electrical, weak or strong nuclear, or magnetic or electromagnetic forces. The information telling a field or force what to do and how to do it can either cause or cure cancer. Conversely, the vibration of and information held within a field can either cause or cure cancer.

Long ago, a researcher named Harold Saxton Burr became convinced that fields actually instruct the body rather than the other way around. He was able to detect cancer in a person's fields before a diagnosis was made, showing that what we pick up energetically can affect our physical health.[7]

One interesting subject in the area of magnetics concerns the effect of "geopathic stress" on our health. Geopathic fields are generated by the natural world. We are all affected by the background of magnetic fields from nature. People are usually healthier in general when they are surrounded by nature; aberrant magnetic fields, however, are dangerous. Geopathic stress zones are caused by electromagnetic fluctuations or abnormal earth fields. Researchers in Germany have shown that living in such zones is linked to a higher than normal rate of cancer. In one project, Ludger Meersman, a geobiology researcher, used special equipment to monitor the magnetic fields around people's beds when they were sleeping. Abnormal magnetic readings "corresponded to the part of the patient's body afflicted with arthritis or cancer."[8] We are affected by what we perceive vibrationally around us.

In addition, we can use vibrational means, such as field treatments, to treat cancer. Early in the twentieth century, G. Lakhovsky used high-frequency fields to treat cancer, as he believed that health required the correct electrical balance in living cells. Recent research is supporting his theories.[9] In yet another study, Dr. Albert Davis and Walter C. Rawls conducted research with magnetic-field stimulation. They "produced significant reductions in tumor growths in animals by exposing them to relatively intense (greater than 2,500 gauss) north magnetic fields."[10] Cancer responds to vibrational healing.

Intensity Intensity has to do with how hard you work to make something happen. On the elemental pathway, you must exert a lot of force to create change. On the divine pathway, force actually creates a negative outcome. You must learn when to push for change and when to just allow change to happen.

Motion Since time began, healers have capitalized on ideas about motion to effect healing. Motion is about movement, which is really about vibration. As discussed in the preceding section on vibration, however, there are countless motions available to any unit of energy. Some motions are beneficial, and some are harmful.

The three chief ingredients of motion in pathway healing are speed, spin, and form.

THE TERM *FORM* HAS SEVERAL MEANINGS IN REGARD TO CHAKRA-BASED healing. Scientifically, the word *form* indicates the nature, structure, or essence of a thing. It also stands for the shape or appearance of something that makes it identifiable. In pathway healing, there are also two types of beings that can be described with the term *forms.* One is a group of entities that can actually transform energies from one nature or shape to another. These are beings most similar to angels, in that they are innately able to perform this task. Second is a group of beings that over time develop the ability to alter energies in this same way. These forms are beings that have become so identified with their craft that they lose physicality and emanate the pure energy of their knowledge. A person can become a form, if he or she masters a craft to this extent. When pairing the term *form* with ideas like motion and speed, I'm referencing the idea of form as shape. The essential energy of a toad, for instance, performs differently when shaped differently. A toad in its early stages of development is a tadpole. Tadpoles have tails, and so they can swim. After transforming shape, the same being now holds a different form, that of a toad. Toads are better at jumping than swimming. Energy workers often play with the shape of energies to produce the desired effects. For instance, you can both analyze and change the forms of an energy for healing, most specifically working with geometric forms, tones, images, and numbers.

Speed is the velocity of energy. We've discussed the ability to move matter faster and slower than the speed of light and to freeze it in place. The ease of determining speed varies among the pathways.

Spin is the configuration of a moving energy. Spin studies have produced a following among physicists, who are now reading spin to determine the nature of an object and ways to control reality. There are two aspects to spin. In the physical plane, for instance, you might see an object spinning in a circle. When working some of the other pathways, specifically the imagination pathway, you have to consider the points of the spin that can't be seen through a third-dimension lens. The points that intersect with other worlds are actually able to gather information and energies to enable healing and are therefore as important as the points that you can see in the third dimension.

Energy on the Pathways

As stated previously, each pathway is an energetic level of a Greater Reality. Negative, positive, and neutral energies exist in each reality; however, you access and use these concepts differently on each pathway.

On the elemental pathway, you must be precise in your use of information, vibration, and motion. The elemental world is a complex and intricate weaving of all sorts of energies. One slip and you could create a disaster. One positive move and you can create great change.

On the power pathway, you have to be deliberate. This is a world of forces, and you can create great change with little effort. You must know what you are doing, however, or you may find yourself accidentally supporting the enemy rather than the allies.

On the imagination pathway, the key is magical thinking. There are worlds beyond this one, and by applying your knowledge of particle typing, fields, forces, speed, spin, and form you can produce miraculous results. To work this pathway, you must ultimately trust your own senses and intuition.

On the divine pathway, there are no mistakes. Cancer is not seen as obscene; it is a lens through which you can better see and understand the nature of love.

How can you most easily apply particle and wave theory for healing? In many ways, this entire book is devoted to answering this question. The short response: by directing little or big energies for change, you can change just about anything. For instance, there is enough explosive strength in a single particle to blow up a mountain. A single thought contains that much potential, as does a feeling, a belief, or a word. Waves from the power pathway can sweep away the most potent of physical walls. Think of what one might do if directed against a cancerous tumor! There are thousands of ways to access the forces of particles and waves, and all of them are available to those who know how to recognize the various forms of energy and marshal them at will. What's needed to become an energy worker of this magnitude? Knowledge, pure and simple.

chapter three

Knowledge: A Power Tool in the Anticancer Tool Kit

i think a wind is blowing up above
but the wind is such a meaningless thing.
invisible and always gone.
i still think it was wind.

—Andrew Clements, *Things Not Seen*[1]

A cancer diagnosis results in fear and confusion. Feeling and expressing our feelings are a critical part of healing, but it's also possible to get lost in our personal reactions to the disease. In this chapter, you are invited to step out of the emotional aspect of cancer long enough to fully engage your mind in the healing process. Knowledge will help you make logical, rational, and effective decisions about your own or another's healing needs.

Knowing What You Need to Know

Knowledge is one of the most important tools for pathway healing.

Knowledge is one of the precursors to wisdom, which also involves applying personal experience to a task. A wise healer first studies the situation at hand and then arrives at a strategy.

First and foremost, you need to understand what cancer is. How can you fight an enemy if you don't know what it looks like? How can you befriend a foe that you don't understand? In this chapter, I review several definitions of cancer, starting with a medical review of the condition. I also interlace perspectives unique to energy and pathway work throughout this discussion, so you can begin to see how the standard ideas of cancer link with pathway philosophies.

Essential to pathway healing is the ability to pinpoint the exact cause of a cancerous condition. There are many theories about how someone gets cancer. To give you the broadest view, I discuss the ideas most frequently offered by traditional and alternative health care providers and then outline the types of causes found when conducting pathway healing. Then onward to healing modalities. As you might expect, there are similarities among the treatments provided by traditional, holistic, and pathway healing, and also variations. After presenting some of the main treatment methods in each category, I then assess each for problems and potentials.

Finally, I have included a short section on the role of fear in healing. Cancer is a scary disease. In most healing methods, fear is seen as an opponent. One crucial difference in pathway healing is that fear is seen as an asset, not a liability. In fact, fear is considered an important power tool for healing. (In the end, almost anything can be transformed into a tool for healing.) Through the pathway process, you learn to use your fear in healthy rather than unhealthy ways.

What Is Cancer from a Medical Point of View?

What is cancer? The word was actually assigned to the condition more than two thousand years ago by the famous Greek philosopher Hippocrates. He used words referencing the crab, like *carcinos* and *carcinoma*, to describe tumors that had fingerlike projections. We now call cancers *carcinomas* and *malignancies*, both terms for describing the incessant and invasive action of a cancer.

Cancer is actually an out-of-control growth of abnormal cells. These abnormal cells proliferate and spread through several stages in a process called *carcinogenesis*. Damage to one or more genes, the controlling programs of the cells, causes abnormal growth. The genes most involved in cancer problems are *oncogenes*, which stimulate growth, and *tumor-suppressor genes*, which prevent cancer except when injured. Current science has isolated one hundred oncogenes and fifteen tumor-suppressor genes, any combination of which can be the cause of a cancerous tumor; this means that each tumor is basically unique.

All cells are designed to die or be destroyed before they pass on mutations or dangerous changes. As a cell ages, its tips, called *telomeres*, become depleted, and the chromosomes on them become unstable. At this point, the cell dies. Except when the cell is a cancer cell. Cancer cells produce an enzyme, *telomerase*, that replaces the lost portion of the tips. Just about any cell can become cancerous, but there are certain cells more prone to cancer than others, for many reasons. Some cells duplicate more often than other cells, which creates more margin for error. Other cells are more heavily used than others and therefore more apt to become injured or inflamed—also key factors in cancer. Regardless, because of their telomerase tips, cancer cells don't die. They now duplicate faster than healthier cells. The daughter cells, as they are called, don't develop into healthy cells. They never mature, and their growth is disorderly. Often this is because of genetic damage. The genes telling the daughter cells how to behave and act have changed through cellular reproduction.

The information inside of a cell is supposed to tell it how to act in an orderly and healthy way. But the information inside cancer cells tells them to be disorderly rather than orderly. If you want to become skilled at pathway healing, remember this point.

Working energetically is about working with information. The malignant cells multiply quickly. As they pile up, these daughter cells and their daughter cells form tumors, which feed off the body's blood supply while choking off normal cells.

Cancer cells eventually destroy surrounding tissue and often spread throughout the body in the process called *metastasizing*. This happens when cancer cells cross normal boundaries and invade other parts of the body. Journeying through the bloodstream or the lymph system, these traveling vagabonds often form secondary tumors. Secondary tumors usually mirror their origination point, the primary tumor. The cancer cells break their way into new territory by producing enzymes that dissolve the cement between healthy cells. Pushing their way in, they take over.

All cancerous tumors block the healthy functioning of the part of the body that they occupy. Some cancer cells also produce substances that are poisonous for the body and affect the muscles, salt regulation, or nerves.

You could say that cancer cells are the cellular equivalent of vampires — humans that should be dead, but aren't. Cancer cells are undead cells that feed off living cells in order to maintain their state.

In short, cancer involves these steps:

1. Mutated genes cause cells to proliferate uncontrollably.
2. These cells refuse to die when they should.
3. The cancer cells spread to tissue where they don't belong.
4. Eventually, these cells choke the life out of healthy cells.

The Importance of Determining a Cancer's Location

If you or a loved one has cancer, I suggest that you learn the medical terms that your professional helpers use for diagnosis, as you'll want to be an informed participant in the decision-making process.

I've noted that the original location of the cancer or the primary tumor is called the *primary site*. In both traditional medical and pathway healing, caregivers usually want to figure out where this site is; they also must determine how far the cancer has progressed, a diagnostic process called *staging*. This information is an essential part of your healing tool kit. By determining the primary site you can pinpoint the causes and therefore the best solutions for that particular cancer. By assessing the stage, you can establish how fast the cancer is spreading and select healing tools based on the time available for your healing work.

Staging determines how much cancer is in the body and where it is located. When undertaking staging, medical professionals assess the advancement of the cancer according to locality. As cancer progresses, it goes through several stages. Most cancers are classified in one of five stages, 0 to IV. In the earlier stages, cancers are small and geographically confined. Later stages involve the spread of cancers to the lymph nodes or elsewhere in the body. Primary site tumors might be in different stages than secondary site tumors. Both types of tumors, however, are usually made of the same basic material.

When conducting pathway healing, you can work the same way in all tumor sites, because the cause and effects will be similar. Most of the time, if you determine which chakra the primary site is in, you address the needs connected with that chakra first. When you do this, sometimes the secondary tumors are taken care of automatically. If not, you then deal with the concerns affecting the secondary tumor site independently.

At times it's difficult to find a primary tumor site. This occurs if the cancer is so widespread that it is impossible to determine the initial location. As well, some cancers are systemic. In these cases, I usually suggest working with the chakra that most often regulates the systems most negatively affected by the cancer, or the chakra(s) that initiates the concerns most affected by the cancer. For instance, a widespread blood cancer influences every area of the body. Blood disorders most often involve the chakras in the groin and the heart areas therefore I would prompt the client to energy map in both of these localities.

There is yet another important term to add to your knowledge tool kit: *grading*. Grading refers to the aggressiveness of the cancer, as studied under a microscope. This is an important feature in treating some cancers, although staging is usually of greatest concern.

What Causes Cancer?

What causes cancer cells to act so irrationally? There are many theories. Here are a few, taken from both the traditional medical and the current holistic models.

Potential Causes of Cancer: Traditional Medical Theories

Traditional doctors and researchers point the finger at these reasons for contracting cancer:

- Genetics
- Smoking
- Alcohol consumption
- Antibiotic use (linked to breast cancer)
- Hormones in meat and milk
- Increased consumption of sugar and white flour
- Environmental toxins
- Additives and food preparation methods
- Sexual and reproductive behavior
- Gender
- Stress
- Radiation exposure

- Sunlight
- Other illnesses, especially those such as AIDS that compromise the immune system
- Use of chemicals and drugs, even medicinally
- Dietary factors and allergies
- Repressed immune system
- Former stresses (seen in correlations between sexual abuse and female genital cancers, for example)

This list merely outlines the types of situations or irritants that might cause cells to mutate. All cancer involves genetic mutation; however, there are several theories about the ways that cancer cells mutate. At this time, there are four major hypotheses to explain the genetic alterations that create cancer.

Standard Dogma According to this theory, various carcinogens — such as tobacco, sunlight, or antibiotics — alter the DNA of affected cells. These mutations cause growth-inhibiting proteins to disappear, so the cells survive when they shouldn't. Mutations to oncogenes stimulate *oncoproteins*, which give the cell superhuman survival skills. The cells form a mass and then some break off, spreading the cancer.

Modified Dogma According to this premise, one or more of the genes needed to repair DNA become disabled. Random mutations occur. Eventually the cancer-related genes take over, and the cancer increases and spreads as described in the standard dogma.

Early Instability This conjecture is based on the concept that some form of stress causes one or more of the "master genes" to become silenced. Chromosomes multiply, but now mistakes occur, getting worse with each generation. Over time, the proteins that suppress tumors decrease, and the cancerous cells take over.

All-Aneuploidy According to this theory, arising from the most recent body of studies, a mistake that occurs during cellular division results in cells with odd numbers of chromosomes, called *aneuploid cells*.

Aneuploid cells are usually destroyed by regular means, but in the beginnings of cancer a few survive and live within body tissue. It may take years or even decades for these cells to spread. What makes these cells proliferate? Somehow, the aneuploid cells acquire the superhuman abilities described by the other standard cancer dogmas. This theory differs from the others, however, in that it suggests that cells become malignant even before the master genes, oncogenes, or tumor suppressor genes mutate.

If the fourth theory is true, then even traditional science must consider new approaches to healing cancer. Tumors always evolve into resistant strains. Traditional approaches seem to merely delay an eventual overgrowth of new cancerous cells. As *Scientific American*'s W. Wayt Gibbs points out, "the best you can hope for is to delay the tumor's growth. You are not going to cure it."[2]

Physical Conditions that Set the Stage

We used to think that as long as we could keep our hearts ticking, we could make it into old age. But cancer has now pulled ahead of heart disease as the leading cause of death among Americans under age eighty-five. We are walking time bombs.

Medical science is postulating that one of the main reasons for the increased rate of cancer over recent decades is the depletion and pollution of the environment. It's a well-known fact that the environment is becoming highly toxic. Industry, factories, cars, powered boats, farms, oil wells, nuclear power sites, power lines, sewage systems, and hundreds of other facilities emit or pump out waste products that end up in the waterways, soils, and air, creating complications that defy a simple solution. Picture the various ways in which we are tearing the web of life outside of our bodies; then imagine how these same conditions affect the inside of our bodies.

Water is our lifeblood. Over 75 percent of the human body is made of water, making it the most important substance that we consume. It is said that we could live on nothing but water for a two-week period. Water is life.

Our bodies are designed to filter waste, our liver and kidneys serving as primary organs in this process. Water then flushes these waste products out of our bodies, primarily through our lungs, skin, and excretory system. When everything clicks, the toxins that we naturally consume and create within our bodies are constantly released, maintaining a healthy and balanced body. What happens when the key to this cleansing process is itself toxic? Daily, tons of pollution and waste enter our oceans and groundwater before being converted to farming and drinking water. Sure, before we drink water we filter and treat it (a process that often adds additional chemicals and substances to the water), but there's no way to manage the seepage and dumping of chemicals and pollutants that make their way into water everywhere.

The effects of toxic water are horrendous. The lethal substances in water clog the body's cleansing systems, decreasing the effectiveness of the liver, kidneys, and lymph and encouraging the storage of toxic by-products in our tissues. Areas of high toxicity eventually become inflamed. Inflammation is one of the major preconditions for the development of cancer cells.

Polluted water also affects animals, fish, and plants and, in turn, distresses us. Lakes, rivers, and oceans have become polluted with various sources of toxins, including farm runoff, industrial dumping, oil seepage, and more. Due to lack of regulations or enforcement, livestock drink water that contains even more noxious toxins than we consume, and they often graze on land full of poisonous fertilizers. What animals consume shows up on the kitchen table. The food of the sea is becoming sewage from the sea.

Water and plant life intersect to compound the damage. Farm land is frequently treated with fertilizer and insecticide sprays. These toxic additives make it into our crops through groundwater and runoff. We consume the resulting grains, fruits, and vegetables, as do food animals, creating a steady influx into our diets of "free radicals" — highly reactive atoms that bombard the body, stressing the immune system and encouraging cell mutation.

We're also poisoning animal feed quite independently of this "accidental watering." Most stock animals are injected with hormones and chemicals to encourage a fast growth rate and lower rate of illness. Antibiotics are given to most flesh animals. Every time you consume meat or dairy products from these animals, you ingest a dose of antibiotics, lowering your resistance to the antibiotic that you might need in the future and furthering the development of resistant strains of bacteria. Studies have linked increased antibiotic consumption to cancers including breast cancer, so women especially should avoid treated dairy products. Milk is further treated with a variety of chemicals that many people insist results in an overstimulation of hormones.

Hormones are a very real factor in the overall increased incidence of cancer. Various studies establish the connection between cancer rates and high estrogen in women and testosterone changes in men. For instance, the more exposure a woman has to estrogen during her lifetime, the greater her chance of developing breast cancer. You're not only drinking your hormones in dairy, you're consuming them in various meats and through compounds in other foods, air, and water supplies.

Hormones are regularly added to the diets of beef cattle and other animals raised for the table, including pigs, sheep, and chickens. There are six hormones typically added to meat. Imagine what occurs inside of your body when it's being pumped with additional estrogen, progesterone, and testosterone-related hormones, as well as the adrenaline that enters an animal's bloodstream when it is being butchered. Many medical experts postulate that the increasingly early age of puberty among children comes from this amplified hormone consumption.

There are demonstrated benefits to avoiding such foods. In my own practice, I see enormous gains in health when women and men shift from hormone- and antibiotic-laced products to grass-fed, organic, natural, free-range, or preservative-free sources. Outcomes include more energy; less illness; better memory and concentration; lowered premenstrual, premenopausal, or menopausal symptoms; augmented libido; and loss of excess weight.

The estrogen-like compounds in chemicals and pesticides also stimulate cancer growth. The body can't recognize the difference between many chemicals and pesticides and estrogen or other hormones; thus it responds as if it is overloaded with estrogen. These substances are sometimes found in ingested substances like produce and water, but are also present in many household products, such as laundry detergents.

Another form of food poisoning is occurring within the packaged food industry. Most fast or processed "convenience" foods are made with trans fats, which increase the rate of cancer and heart disease in the human body. These foods are also loaded with sugar, which decreases immune function, an important defense against the development and spread of cancer. Sugar consumption also encourages tissue inflammation and diabetes; diabetics have an increased risk of developing both circulatory problems and cancer. Unhealthy fats, sugars, and chemical additives and preservatives establish the ground for cell mutation and also take the place of the vegetables, whole grains, fruits, and healthy fats that inhibit the start or spread of cancer.

One human resource shared by all is the air. What's in the air enters the lungs, moving from the lungs to your blood vessels, from the blood to your organs, and then to the inner workings of your cells. Inhale healthy air, and you have healthier cells; unhealthy air results in unhealthy cells. Car emissions alone are enough to choke most of us, but consider also the effects of two other types of air pollution.

Smoking is the number one controllable factor in preventing cancer. It increases your chance of getting cancer — especially lung cancer — by a dozen times over. In fact, 90 percent of all people with lung cancer have smoked at some time in their lives. And smokers can directly pollute nonsmokers' airways: "secondhand smoke" increases its victims' chances of getting cancer by upward of 50 percent.

Another frequently overlooked form of air pollution is the constant barrage of emissions from power plants, communications devices, electrical facilities, nuclear sites, and even products right in the kitchen, such as microwaves. We've all read about the fallout of nuclear devastation, such as that experienced in World War II in Japan and later in Chernobyl in the Soviet Union. Radiation causes cancer; I have had several Russian clients who, exposed to Chernobyl, died years later of various forms of cancer. We tend to overlook the long-term effects of these and other radiation and electromagnetic sources, including those that emanate from former nuclear explosions or tests, geomagnetic or soil sources, and even luxury appliances.

Yes, even your kitchen appliances can create the conditions for cancer! After all, they are electrical, and anything electrical can potentially warp your own electromagnetic field.

Think of your body as an electrical device. Your heart generates 50,000 times more electricity than does your brain; it must do so to maintain the integrity of your body, the structure of your organs, the inner workings of your cells, the generation of cells in your bone marrow, and the magnetic frequency that surrounds your body, serving as a protective shield. Any significant shift in electricity or magnetism around your body, and your heart and central nervous system will respond adversely, thus compromising the function of every single part of your body — including the functions in the nucleus of your cells.

Various studies are revealing the devastating effects of exposure to warped electromagnetism. There is a significant rise in the incidence of cancer in people living near power plants, for instance, or those exposed to long-range missile sites. The viability of your cells depends on several factors. When the electromagnetic balance is thrown off, the cell cannot maintain its own integrity, and genetic mutation can be one of the results.

Basically, toxicity from the environment and diet encourages genetic defects or the mutation of cells due to free-radical damage. If our immune system can't keep up with the inflow or buildup of free radicals or toxins at large, then cells mutate, becoming cancerous.

One of the main defenses against free radicals — and therefore against cancer — is the antioxidant. Antioxidants cleanse the body of free radicals, thus protecting us against cancer. Our major source of antioxidants is food, especially fruits and vegetables. Unfortunately, environmental poisoning and the resulting changes in soil are making it more and more challenging to derive antioxidants from our diets. Breast cancer patients, for instance, are shown to have low levels of the antioxidants selenium, glutathione, vitamin C, vitamin E, bioflavonoids, carotenoids, and coenzyme Q10 — substances not found in artificially produced foods or those grown in depleted soil. Decreased levels of selenium, for instance, are directly related to the development of breast, liver, and prostate cancers. Our soils have been stripped of selenium due to years of inadequate farming procedures and increased consumption of packaged foods instead of selenium-rich products such as nuts and vegetables.

Consider also the role of the antioxidant glutathione in the battle against cancer. Glutathione protects and regulates a tumor suppression protein involved in over half of all cancers. This protein gives the body time to repair any DNA damage before cell division can multiply a cancer cell, and in some cancer cells it can completely stop cell division, thereby destroying the cancer. But this protein works only in the presence of glutathione, which is difficult to obtain in the current American diet.

Why is cancer overwhelming our society? On the physical level, it looks like we're doing it to ourselves.

Potential Causes of Cancer: Holistic Theories

According to most holistic models, serious diseases like cancer have mental, emotional, or spiritual causes, in addition to physical ones — causes such as these:

- Repressed feelings
- Inaccurate beliefs
- Lack of faith in a higher being
- Hopelessness
- Karma, or problems from the past
- Original sin: God's punishment for others' sins
- Others' energies
- Psychic invasion
- Spiritual choices

To this list, holistic practitioners would add the causes of cancer covered by traditional medical thinkers. However, an alternative care provider would insist on looking underneath the presenting symptoms or physical issues for emotional, mental, spiritual, or even energetic reasons for cancer.

Several studies have pointed out that repressed feelings can lead to major illnesses such as cancer. Research by Lydia Temoshok, Ph.D., at the University of Maryland School of Medicine and through the Behavioral Medicine program at the Institute of Human Virology shows that cancer spreads faster in patients who don't recognize or act on their feelings. Temoshok believes that emotional withholding increases stress hormones, which in turn depress the immune system and accelerate the progression of cancer.[3]

Since the 1980s, a series of studies has revealed the connection between beliefs and illnesses. Negative, morose, and pessimistic people get ill more frequently and die sooner of their illnesses. There's a similar pattern in relationship with faith.

Documentation shows that people who believe in a higher power and attend a place of worship get ill less frequently, recover sooner, and have a lower incidence of death from a contracted major illness within a certain time frame than do their nonpraying, nonchurchgoing counterparts.

When entering the world of energy, you open the door to even more potential causes of cancer. Many people believe in reincarnation — the idea that you have lived other lives before your current one. Issues carried over from a former incarnation can be the reason for contracting an illness in this lifetime.

The explanation of reincarnated problems is founded on the belief that patterns linger from lifetime to lifetime. You might have a greater chance of contracting and dying from lung cancer in this lifetime, for instance, if you worked in a coal mine and died from cancer in a former incarnation. When born anew, the bodily weakness from the former incarnation becomes locked into your current body. Another slant on the theory is that certain people might become afflicted with cancer as a "payback" for sins from another time period. Let's say you were the owner of a coal mine in a former life and were therefore responsible for the deaths of hundreds of workers. Your current cancer condition might originate in a soul or spiritual contract, in which you agreed to experience the pain and agony that you previously put others through.

This way of thinking — often referred to in spiritual circles as a belief in karma, or retributive justice — suggests a positive reason for getting cancer. Perhaps your soul has chosen the disease as a way of learning. Before wondering why anyone would want cancer, consider the valuable life lessons provided by the disease. Cancer can point out the importance of caring for the body, the preciousness of life itself, the imminence of death, the desire for relationship, the interdependence of humans and the environment, and the depths of compassion and charity.

One striking study, conducted by Dr. Joel Whitton, professor of psychiatry at the University of Toronto Medical School, revealed a potential connection between decisions made before birth and the tragedies of today. After being hypnotized, study subjects disclosed memories of other times and events, many of which explained issues, like phobias, that affect them in their current lives. Most striking in relation to our discussion about cancer are the regressions conducted to the time period in between lives, which the subjects experienced as a dazzling, light-filled realm; hence in my own work I have come to name this space the *white zone*. Whitton found that his subjects entered a depth of knowing that he called "metaconsciousness," a state of heightened moral and ethical awareness. When preparing for their upcoming lives, the souls in this state often agreed to life events that would teach them lessons, sometimes to include a serious illness. One individual rewrote the script and, when still conducting sessions with Whitton, experienced a near-miraculous and complete recovery.[4]

Yet another, more religious rationale for cancer is founded in the belief in original sin. According to Jewish, Islamic, and all Christian doctrines, humans sinned against God while in the Garden of Eden and have thus been condemned to the punishment of pain, suffering, illness, and death. Within this viewpoint is the rationale for the existence of cancer: simply by being human, you are born in a state of darkness and are thus prone to the wiles of evil, which include deadly diseases like cancer. Although you might not be personally responsible for the sins underlying cancer, you are genetically and morally susceptible.

People who understand energy, myself included, toss another suggestion into the cancer-causing basket: energetics. We are all made of energy. Energy can flow in psychic and fast forms or sensory and slow forms. Fast-moving energy has no boundaries. It can pass right through your skin (an organ) and even through cellular walls. Once converted from fast- to slow-moving energy, which is possible through the chakras and other energy bodies, a psychic package can solidify into a form that can either assist or interfere with the body's normal processes. Someone else's critical thoughts, disease patterns, repressed feelings, or even toxic wastes can thus enter your bloodstream and clog your lymph system. The buildup of these negative intruders can then congeal as waste products, which induces inflammation. In reaction, the body might build cyst or tumor walls to encapsulate the toxins. Over time, the material within this walled-off fort mutates, creating cancer.

There are many other holistic theories as to the cause of cancer, which of course also embrace the practical, such as environmental poisoning and dietary malnutrition. These ideas, in total, invite exposure to worldviews that can only benefit the person on the cancer journey. The more open your mind, the more solutions you might find.

Potential Causes of Cancer: Pathway Approach

There are thousands of ways to look at cancer through the lens of the Four Pathways approach. This is partly because the pathway process embraces a considerable number of traditional and holistic theories about the causes of cancer. The main distinction is that on the pathways you search for causes in many levels of reality and within these in many other subareas. This thoroughness increases your chances of pinpointing an exact cause for a cancerous condition. Even on the more physical of all pathways, the elemental, you will consider causes beyond those noted by traditional or holistic philosophies.

This array of choices can be confusing. Remember that we're dealing with cancer. Each person is unique. Each cancer is unique. To really heal from cancer, you absolutely must consider the assortment of causal factors. Know that there is probably one main cause for your cancer or that of a loved one, and perhaps up to a hundred other factors that branch off of the core reason.

Throughout this book, you'll be taught a variety of ways to isolate the major possible reason that you have cancer in your life.

Let's look at some of the potential causes of cancer, as seen on each of the Four Pathways.

The Elemental Pathway

On the elemental pathway, all cancer reduces to a physical cause. You might consider the list of traditional medical causes provided earlier in this chapter, as well as the more emotional, mental, and spiritual issues added by various holistic philosophies. However, to achieve full healing on the elemental pathway you will probably have to dig a little deeper, into the world of quantum physics and energy.

At baseline, all cancers on the elemental pathway downgrade to errant vibrations or information or the combination, informed vibration. We will be examining this statement in more depth throughout this book and particularly in chapter 4, but for now know this: each cell has an optimum vibration, which is determined in part by the information within and around it. When physical or psychic energies of a different vibration overpower a healthy cell, the core information of that cell can become compromised. What matter carries the baseline information that tells a cell how to be and operate? The genes. Bad information or vibration disrupts your genes and causes cancer.

There are countless energies that endanger the informed vibration of your healthy cells. When working the elemental pathway, you want to get rid of the invading marauders and alter the energetics so that cells can return to a normal state of fluctuation and functioning. If this fails to work, you might need to help the body recognize the malignant cells so that your immune system can wipe them out. To accomplish these and other goals, you work elementally by examining for three basic types of energies: negative, positive, or neutral. You then review physical factors for a more direct diagnosis, searching for problems in areas including the environment, elements, exercise, diet, symbology, interference, feelings, thoughts, spiritual principles, and various spacetimes and other planes of existence.

The Power Pathway

The power pathway is a sea of endless energies and powers. There are limitless forces at play in this realm, but most are either destructive or constructive. The self on the power pathway might be accessing and using these various energies quite appropriately, which provides for almost superhuman health and strength. Besides energies, there are also beings that subsist on this pathway that can provide helpful insight and advice. On the other hand, mistaken notions and beliefs, childhood experiences and family patterns, and soul issues and damage can cause the "power self" to misuse the power forces; this can lead to all sorts of life problems, including disease.

Lack of knowledge about the power pathway and its energies can result in disastrous consequences. You can't correctly use a power that you don't know anything about. Sometimes our subconscious or unconscious will align with power forces in a way that is detrimental, thinking that it is doing you a favor. Misinformed application of forces can easily cause or reinforce a cancer, even if the goal was to enable health.

I look to the power pathway for causal diagnosis when a cancer strikes swiftly or suddenly, when a cancer "should" be healed according to contemporary wisdom but isn't disappearing, or when a cancer appears throughout a family group. In all likelihood, the supernatural forces available for health on the power pathway are instead supporting disease.

There is yet another indication of power problems. The power pathway is a world unto itself, but often the energies of this plane bleed onto other pathways, usually the elemental. If I've pinpointed a cancer on the elemental pathway but it's not responding to elemental treatments, I then look to the power pathway to see if any of its energies are "plugged into" elemental properties, thus sustaining the physical cause of a cancer. The cause of these cancers isn't technically power-based, but power forces are keeping the cancer alive and so must be addressed.

The Imagination Pathway

We can imagine our way to health, but the opposite is also true. Through the imagination, you have direct access to any and all possibilities, including a future completely devoid of cancer. This and other potential futures exist in the antiworld that occupies the imagination pathway. As well, futures involving the spread of, debilitation from, or death from cancer are also available through the imagination pathway.

On the imagination pathway, I look for cancers that are caused by the choices that lead to cancer. We might unconsciously think that we deserve cancer, or that because our mother died of cancer, so must we. We could volunteer to "make a point" about the dangers of environmental toxicity by allowing our imagination to construct cancer. Essentially, cancer on the imagination pathway is caused by the belief that it is our only choice for the accomplishment of a certain goal — or that it is the only choice, period.

The Divine Pathway

Cancer on the divine pathway is recognized as a question to which the only answer is love. It is simply an attempt to receive, give, or understand love, even if the process doesn't seem self-loving from a human viewpoint.

As divine beings having a human experience called "life," we entered this world to learn more about love. If at some level we believe that the only way to acquire a certain teaching about love is to contract cancer, our body responds by getting cancer. Love doesn't cause cancer on the divine pathway; the perceived lack of love causes the cancer.

When working on the divine pathway, you will determine which of seven basic lies or untruths has led to a misunderstanding about love. It's difficult to place our faith in divine or human love when badness seems to run the earth. Eventually, we each must come to terms with these seven lies or illusions by asking ourselves if the persistence of difficulties really negates the truth of love or not. Cancer (or any of a number of other diseases and problems) may come from believing that one of these lies is greater than the truth of the Greater Reality.

Potential Causes of Cancer from an Intelligent Energy Point of View

All energy is intelligent. That's because all energy contains information. Your cancer cells might seem stupid; after all, how long will they survive if they eliminate their host? Cancer cells don't worry about their long-range survival, however. The core programming that ensured cell viability and integrity has been wiped out. Although they might not pass the standard IQ tests, cancer cells are smart enough to get rid of the competition, take over the country that is your body, and reign supreme.

There are three main agendas or intelligence programs that create and sustain cancer. You could say that there are three main types of cancers, and that all cancers fall into one of these categories. Here basic physics is at play in your body, in that all physical matter reduces to charges that are electrical, magnetic, or inert. Thus cancer is fundamentally either (1) an electron-based or electrical condition, (2) a proton-based or magnetic condition, or (3) a neutron-based or neutral condition. Here are the three main types of cancer from an information-energy perspective.

Electron-Based Cancers

Electrons hold negative charges, which are electrical. Cancers can be caused by having too many negative charges collected in one area, which distorts the normal flow of electrical energy in the body, the fields around the body, and, over time, the programming of intracellular DNA.

How does this happen? Electrons hold information that is chiefly emotional, physical, and psychic in nature. Their job is enabling you to be powerful. Electrons also maintain the body's structure, even down to insisting that your DNA stays orderly and that your cellular walls hold steady. When situations occur that decrease your ability to act or be powerful, the resultant unexpressed feelings and beliefs get stored in the electrons in your physical and energetic system. Your structures go awry. This data is gathered by your subconscious and sometimes your unconscious and is used by your energy system to relate this information to the world.

There are several in-body chakras, all of which link to your spine. These chakras transmit sensory and psychic information between your brain, your central nervous system, and the rest of your body, as well as the nonphysical aspects of yourself. When negatively stored issues, beliefs, and feelings become too heavy or intrusive, the chakras cannot function well. Dysfunctional chakras create many effects, including a warping of your electrical system — the electricity generated primarily by your heart and secondarily by your brain to manage bodily functions. Conversely, injuries in the neurological or electrical system are borne by the chakras, which then can't meet the demands laid upon them.

How can "bad feelings" create cancer? We can understand that the chemical or electrical emanations from radiation, poisons, or toxins can affect DNA changes, but feelings? Specific research, as explained by Doc Lew Childre in his book *Freeze Frame*, uses an electrocardiogram analysis to show that difficult emotions including hostility, frustration, worry, and anxiety adversely affect the electrical patterns of the heart. In comparison, emotions such as love, care, and compassion have positive effects.[5] Positive feelings coordinate the vibrations of respiration, heart rate, and pulse transit time, creating what is called a "coherent spectrum." Electrical energy is radiated to every cell in your body. Negative or challenging feelings and beliefs are expressed throughout your entire system and disrupt the body's mechanisms, eventually causing decay within your cells.

Scientific researchers like Dr. Candace Pert are exposing the mechanics of feelings and the ways in which the organic matter of feelings affects the body positively or adversely. As explored in Dr. Pert's book, *Molecules of Emotion,* and the movie *What the Bleep Do We Know?* the brain's programmed reactions to events produce chemical responses in the body. At first, we have simply reacted. Our reactions then stir biochemical activity in the hypothalamus that results in the production of neuropeptide chains. Peptides are proteins, and these neuropeptides are of various lengths and sequential arrangements. Each of the twenty or so types of neuropeptides qualifies as a feeling.

Upon leaving the hypothalamus, the flood of neuropeptides enters the bloodstream. These feeling molecules swarm throughout the body, looking for cells receptive to their chemical programs. Every cell in the body is covered with thousands of receptor sites. If a receptor site is unoccupied, a neuropeptide can enter, much like a key inserting into a lock. The neuropeptide stimulates chemical changes in the cellular wall and in the cell itself, all the way to the nucleus.

Your cells get accustomed to certain neuropeptides. If you are constantly angry, for instance, certain cells become "addicted" or used to the anger molecules. Over time, the constant presence of these invasive proteins can cause damage in the nucleus and therefore in the cell's DNA. As these receiver cells divide, their daughter cells are "born" with the same amount of receptor sites for anger as on the parent sites. One cell with a hundred out of a thousand of its receptor sites addicted to anger now splits into two cells with a hundred out of a thousand receptor sites addicted to anger. All three cells will continue to attract anger neuropeptides.

Let's say that at some point you've collected a ball of one thousand cells, each with seven hundred receptor sites occupied by anger neuropeptides. Guess what? There's scarcely room on these cells for vital vitamins or minerals, or to release intracellular toxins. Receptor sites are the entryways for healthy nutrients and the exit points for waste products. If the receptor sites are occupied by feelings, they can't function in a life-enhancing manner. The ecosystem inside of that cell becomes dark and murky, malnourished and clogged with waste products. Think of the potential DNA damage at this point! If a key telomere or oncogene goes awry, you have conceived cancer. Given that the tissues surrounding this cell are also toxic and affected by malnutrition, the immune system isn't going to perceive the single cancerous cell growing in the muddied waters of thousands of other unhealthy cells.

The inner life of a cell is rich and diverse. One little change in the environment inside or outside of the cell can have drastic effects. Feelings never expressed go somewhere: right into your cells, where they turn the cells into dismal factories of carcinogenic material. As energetic scientific research is now showing, there are few boundaries between cellular parts, including the genetic material. In addition, there is space within the cell that is open to outside influence. The entire living matrix is "mechanical, vibrational or oscillatory, energetic, electronic and informational" at the same time.[6] What you think affects your genes. What you feel affects your genes. What you don't think or feel affects your genes as well.

Distorted electrons, negative charges, and electrical patterns can create cancer. But what does this have to do with the lists of causes provided earlier in this chapter, such as the medical theories? Review the medical list in particular. What do all the factors have in common? Each theory insists that cancer is caused by mutated information. Whether the mistaken data affects the oncogenes, tumor suppression genes, or the basic structure of what becomes an aneuploid cell, data determines structure. A cell cannot hold its correct cellular structure unless the internal information source is telling it to do so, and unless the external environment supports good health.

Proton-Based Cancers

Protons are positively charged. Positive charges are the basis of magnetics, although electrical currents produce magnetic fields. Cancers can be caused by magnetic-based issues that affect the body's ability to function. Conversely, cancer can be cured by magnetic fields and energies.

Protons carry information that is spiritual in nature. Their job is to spread intelligence that allows you to know your divinity and special spiritual abilities. As life unfolds, many of us lose our ability to perceive truth, and we create or take on beliefs that are false. A simple belief — like "I am bad," for instance — if applied to our spiritual nature can keep our body from generating the magnetic energies necessary to clear cancer or any other disease, for that matter. Most proton-based beliefs are unconscious in origin.

Every chakra is affected by your core spiritual beliefs. Believing that sex is evil, for instance, causes restriction in the first chakra, the battery of life energy. When low on life energy, your body runs down. At baseline, your immune system becomes deficient. A healthy immune system is able to prevent the triggering of cancer within aneuploid cells or to kill cancer cells that do develop. If you are repressing the energy needed to support your immune system, you are allowing the gradual development of cancer.

Protons or positively charged conditions are incontestably related to the conditions that cause cancer, as seen in research covered by Phillip Day in his books on alternative healing. On the elemental pathway, electrons are often linked with viral conditions. On this same pathway, proton problems are related to fungal, yeast, or bacterial growth. Research reported by Day is substantiating a higher incidence of cancer where there is an internal growth of fungus or yeast, and in parts of the body most susceptible to these microbes. According to Day, use of substances that kill these microbes and elimination of foods such as sugars from the diet both have a positive effect on the occurrence and healing of cancer.[7] One reason that so many alternative practitioners prescribe gluten-, dairy-, and sugar-free diets is the link between positive charges and beliefs and the physical body. We will discuss one of these diets in chapter 6.

Neutron-Based Cancers

Neutrons are the heaviest of the basic particles, and, although neutrally charged, they are loaded with information. Scientists have suggested that neutrons are the basis of manifestation. First, neutrons gather around an idea. If there are enough neutrons sharing the same data, these neutrons then attract electrons and protons, the remainder of the quotient needed to create physical reality. Conceivably, certain cancers can be caused by mistaken ideas held in the neutrons. In such cases, you can get rid of cancer by reprogramming the cancer-causing or cancer-enhancing data.

The potency of neutrons is indisputable. Research in Russia is showing that through methods similar to fusion, the neutrons of gold can be given indescribable power. Why aren't the Russians pursuing this avenue, originally examined for warfare? They can't direct the forces. The neutron-released strength explodes iron. All human bodies hold iron; therefore, the neutron charges would instantly kill everyone around them. This illustration shows the untapped potential of neutron healing, although I don't recommend that we attempt to discharge our neutrons on this level!

In regard to cancer, I often use the neutron and corresponding state of neutrality on the imagination and divine pathways. On the imagination pathway, you can most easily exchange an unhealthy belief for a healthy belief and see quick change. On the divine pathway, you simply summon forward the love-based belief already held within your spirit, and you automatically open to potent and powerful healing beliefs. I also examine for neutron-based issues on the elemental pathway, as you will treat these cancers somewhat differently than electron- or proton-based cancers, in terms of practical matters like diet.

Available Therapies

There are many therapies available for cancer, ranging from approaches considered medically sound, including chemotherapy and drugs, to those that require a trip to Mexico, such as laetrile injections. In my opinion, you should never substitute an unsubstantiated procedure for a tried and true conventional medical treatment. If you are going to search outside of the box, use alternative methods as supplements, not as mainstays, and then do so only if the procedure doesn't countermand your primary care.

There are many reasons that I make this statement. First, many of the conventional methods work, at least for some people. It's important to follow procedures that have scientific support, as well as professional backing. Not only can you receive the best possible care, but you are also tracked through the traditional system, where you might become a candidate for newer and possibly very effective treatments available on a trial basis. Second, remaining within the acceptable system invites the power of belief. Belief is one of the strongest determinants of outcome. Seeing a doctor who believes in the employed method, surrounding yourself with people who do the same, and aligning with the paradigm already programmed within you by your culture can be good medicine. It's okay to remain locked within the boundaries of your known universe. A few weeks after being diagnosed with lung cancer, my father called and gently informed me that while my "alternative views" probably held merit for my clients, he would put his trust in his oncologist and

God. I completely understood and supported his decision – although I confess to giving him a box of green tea, known to be a lung antioxidant, to serve as a substitute for one of his several cups of black coffee a day.

Many people are dismayed at the process or side effects of conventional treatments. If you question the traditional path, there are already cracks in your belief system or programming. Potentially, your doubts could affect the effectiveness of a standardized treatment. Whether you select any or all recommended conventional treatments, you are a likely candidate to also consider other healing modalities, such as those recommended by alternative care providers or as outlined in the Four Pathways system.

Let's look at some of the therapies available in every mode of medicine, including traditional, holistic, and pathways. I'll offer comparisons of effectiveness, so you can make a more informed choice for yourself or a loved one with cancer.

Traditional Treatments for Cancer

Following are a list of the typical cancer treatments provided by modern Western medicine and an assessment of their effectiveness.

The Standard Traditional Cancer Treatments

The four major conventional treatments are surgery, radiotherapy, chemotherapy, and biologic therapy. Surgery is often employed to cut out the primary tumor and the lymph nodes already infected with cancer. Radiotherapy directs radioactivity to kill the cancer cells. Chemotherapy is the use of chemicals to eliminate cancer cells that exist in the primary and secondary sites. In biologic therapy, medicines and drugs are given to cancer patients as therapy and during recovery.

Problems and Potential of Traditional Care

One of the problems with traditional care, as summarized in a *Fortune* article written in 2004, is that the monies spent on research and development aren't aimed correctly. Scientific and funded research is aimed at shrinking localized tumors — not the smartest goal when 90 percent of deaths from cancer are caused by metastasis, or the spread of cancer.[8] Little research is being done on how to stop the spread of cancer.

However, a hopeful sign is that in recent years modern medicine has finally decided that prevention and early detection might be a more helpful emphasis than treatment of established cancers. There are statistics supporting the benefits of prevention and early detection screening for nearly every type of cancer. Annual check-ups, monthly breast exams, and other early detection techniques can help you spot cancer when it is still relatively easy to treat. Largely due to the introduction of the Pap smear, a test for changes in the cervical cells, the number of deaths from cervical cancer was reduced 74 percent between 1955 and 1992. In men, the death rate from prostate cancer has significantly fallen over the years due to earlier detection as well as a wider range of treatments. Some cancers, such as most childhood leukemia, now have a 90 percent cure rate. And educating the public on the factors within their control — such as diet, sexual partners, exercise and fitness, and regular health exams — has reduced cancer rates and increased the odds of it being detected early.

Typical Holistic Cancer Treatments

There are hundreds — if not thousands — of holistic cancer treatments. I list a few of them along with an analysis of their effectiveness.

Representative Holistic Cancer Treatments

Alternative treatments include adjunctive psychological approaches, such as psychotherapy; imagery, group therapy, and cancer support groups; macrobiotics; nutritional-metabolic programs and various diets, supplements, and herbal treatments; traditional Chinese medicine; religious, energetic, and spiritual healing; technological treatments such as the use of computer, light frequency, and vibrational technologies; electromagnetic therapies; psychic treatment; homeopathy and other vibrational medicines; manipulative treatments such as chiropractic and massage; folk and shamanic treatments; and unconventional therapies such as laetrile, Hoxley herbs, psychoimmunology, or immunosupportive therapies.

Potential and Problems of Alternative Care

Where science sees disease, the alternative practitioner attempts to look for imbalances that need correction. Where the mainstream medical provider notices pain, the alternative care provider tries to assess reasons for the problem. Where traditionalists assess the odds, integrative specialists look at the person.

Some of these approaches work some of the time, but none can be counted upon to work all or even most of the time. As summarized by Michael Lerner in his book, *Choices in Healing*, there seems "no decisive and scientifically documented cure for any type of cancer among the complementary cancer therapies."[9]

The problem is that each person is different. One person's cancer might be caused by repressed feelings, another's by environmental conditions. Alternative medicine is a hunt-and-peck process, and although it can increase your sense of personal power, it can also significantly amplify your frustration.

Pathway Cancer Treatment

Pathway treatments can include any and all traditional and holistic care systems. In the Four Pathways system, you always employ standard procedures, supplementing with other procedures. In fact, if you were using chemotherapy, you would assess the Four Pathways healing tool kit for methods that would enhance rather than detract from the chemotherapy.

The following are a few of the methods for healing cancer used on the pathway approach, an illustration of how these work together, and an assessment of their use and potential effectiveness.

Healing Actions through the Four Pathways Approach

As described in this book — and in *Advanced Chakra Healing: Energy Mapping* — your Four Pathways healing process includes the following methods:

Elemental pathway: Shifting particles and waves; releasing interference; searching for causes in multiple spacetimes; using symbols, colors, numbers, shapes, and tones; dealing with feelings, emotions, and beliefs or other fixations; working with kundalini, elements, pH balance, nutrition, diet, exercise, and other body needs from an energetic perspective; working aspects of the self; ultimately, attaining a neutral state through the chakras and other energy bodies. On the elemental pathway, the emphasis is on supporting the other treatments professionally recommended and monitored by your doctor or health care provider.

Power pathway: Shifting and enhancing spiritual energetic forces through the chakras and their counterparts, the seals. The seals are energy organs that attach to each chakra. They are shaped like lenses. When activated, the concave bowl of a seal receives spiritual energies from the universe, which you can direct through the convex side to focus power for personal use. Activating your seals and using them consciously enables you to aim incredibly potent energies at will. What if you could spotlight a tumor and clarify its cause? Pull a trigger and blast a tumor out of existence? Surround an unhealthy cell with loving healing energy? These are only a few of the potential ways that you can use the seals when working with cancer. If you are already undergoing standard treatment, these powers are used to enhance your therapies and support your body in achieving a balanced state.

Imagination pathway: Shifting energies from the antiworld to this world and vice versa, through the center of a chakra; using symbols to hold new changes; ultimately, achieving a neutral space within a chakra center so you can make healing decisions. The imagination employs creative magic so you can bolster current methods of treatment and support your body in making quick shifts toward health.

Divine pathway: Activating a spiritual wave or quality of truth that combats one of the seven major lies; ultimately, accepting divine love and grace.

Commonalities among the Four Pathways

Though your approach and procedures for healing cancer differ from pathway to pathway, in essence you are always working with three main ideas:

- Information
- Vibration
- Motion

The easiest way to grasp this concept is to picture a simple cell. I'm going to show you how a healthy cell transforms into a cancer cell from the pathway perspective, and how a pathway healing might use information, vibration, and motion to heal from the resulting malignancy.

Let's enter Ted's liver and meet one of Ted's liver cells. We'll call this cell "Larry." Larry, like all his neighbor liver cells, vibrates at a certain frequency or oscillation, one that corresponds to the frequencies of his fellow liver cells and Ted's liver as a whole, and in concert with the chakra that serves all of Ted's digestive organs. Larry is not a spleen cell, and he wouldn't want to be taken for one. No, Susie the spleen cell and her friends are definitely "cut from a different cloth" (and probably use lipstick). All cells vibrate at rates that correspond to their locality, function, and purpose, and Larry is happy about this. He likes being a liver cell.

Larry's vibration is determined in part by the information coded within him. Some of this information emanates from his genes. His genes tell the subatomic particles zipping inside and outside of him how to make him a great liver cell. They inform the molecules inside of him how and when to perform his tasks and keep his cellular walls strong. There are hundreds of other sources of information that tell Larry how to be a top-notch liver cell, such as brain waves, the neuropeptides created in response to emotions, and the informed vibrations of his fellow liver cells. Larry is happy.

But Ted is doing something stupid. Ted eats an enormous amount of bad fats. He does this every time he's mad at someone; he has since he was a child. Larry hates the Bad Fats gang. If he could label their vibration and information, Larry would say that they are big and mean, and they yell at him. They disturb Larry's vibration, and he can't think around them. In the end, he and all his fellow liver cells start moving in the wrong directions. They know that they should hold their own, but the Bad Fats gang makes them sick, and in turn they start making Ted feel sick.

It would all be okay if Ted would listen to Larry and his friends. They shout at Ted, "Hey, you have an upset stomach!" But Ted doesn't listen; in fact, he never has. Larry has a really bad feeling about all of this. Ted should at least be scared, but all that anger and rage keeps Ted from feeling the problem growing inside of his liver. Ted simply continues getting angrier and angrier and eating more and more bad fats. Larry's not sure what he hates worse: the members of the Bad Fat gang or the

Angry Neuropeptides from Ted's hypothalamus that are moving into Larry's neighborhood as if it's a buyer's market in real estate.

It's a gang war, and the Bad Fats are winning.

One day, the Bad Fats finally overpower Larry and his crew. The screaming penetrates all the way into the genetics. The codes that make Larry tick and do his job well start to erode. Larry can feel his programming disintegrate, but he can't do anything about it. It's been so long since he had the support of the Good Fat troupe, he has no vavoom left. Larry sinks into his moroseness, and it's all over. As he falls apart, his body splits into two. His DNA duplicates, but big chunks of it have changed or are missing. Larry is no longer Larry. He is a cancerous cell; in fact, he has become two cancerous cells.

Larry keeps duplicating. There's nothing he can do about it. Pretty soon, the tiny bit of the real Larry within each of his son cells notices that his fellow neighbors are also starting to alter. They, too, have become cancer cells. Is anyone doing anything about this?

Here comes the Four Pathways healer!

The pathways healer assesses the situation, first by figuring out the primary cancer site. She uses vibrational means to do this, but also considers the medically viable origin of the cancer. The data-gathering encompasses knowledge about both the primary chakra site and the primary causal organ. As an intelligent pathway healer, she can derive a lot of data from just these two facts, including knowledge of the potential beliefs, feelings, and core physical anomalies that might have caused the cancer. Our pathway healer will now center in on Larry and his fellow functionaries. What made Bob and his friends get off track? What information, and from what sources, made Larry unhealthy? What other vibrations affected Larry so adversely?

Aha! thinks the healer. *We're dealing with Ted's anger, resentment, and diet.* At this point, our healer is working the elemental pathway exclusively, searching for physical factors. She might decide to move up the pathway scale for a while, traveling through the third chakra as if it were an elevator to take from pathway to pathway. Up one level, she might find that a power force is feeding Ted's anger. Through the imagination pathway, she might determine that Ted made a choice in childhood to repress rather than express his anger, thus shutting off a very real part of his personality in an antiworld. On the divine pathway, our healer learns that Ted thinks that it's loving to hide anger from a loved one, even if it's detrimental to himself.

Having performed this perfunctory diagnosis, our pathway physician now conducts healing in accordance with Ted's selected treatment program. On the elemental pathway, she'll figure out if the cancer is electrical, magnetic, or neutral, then create a protocol. After deciding she's dealing with an electrical issue, she might use regression to help Ted remember the life experiences that established his harmful beliefs about anger. She might insist that he consult with a nutritionist to change his diet. She might assess the elemental properties in his system, even work with an elemental being as an assistant.

"Okay, Ted," she then says. "If you're going to have chemotherapy, let's make sure that it works." She attaches a destructive power force to the chemicals used by Ted's doctors, to bolster their effectiveness. She links a constructive power force to the supplements provided by Ted's alternative care provider, to enhance their efficacy as well. It may be too late for Larry, but can she help the Immune Brothers and Ted's still-healthy liver cells keep their informed vibration at a high level? She moves power forces around to accomplish these goals.

Now our healer might move on to the imagination pathway. "Look, Ted!" she says. "There's an entirely different life path available to you!" Using regression or futuring techniques, she helps Ted figure out how he got into this predicament in the first place and then shows him how to use his own creative magic to make new choices.

Finally, our healer might move Ted onto the divine pathway. "Ted," she queries, "how is this cancer meeting a need for love?"

As Ted ponders the question, he comes to realize that he simply wants to be accepted for who he is. He's not really mad at his wife, his friends, or anyone else; he's really mad at himself for not believing in himself and his own feelings. This epiphany, along with others, invigorates Ted's transformation.

It's too late for Larry. He's now washed out of the system—with a hurrah from the newly created, healthy liver cells. But there's a Laura liver cell in there now, who is programmed with new information — information that is self-loving, self-motivating, and forgiving in nature. She'll never be a cancer cell — no thank you! She's not afraid of any of the big bully Bad Fats that might, once in a while, creep into Ted's diet. Because Ted's not getting angry so often, he's not even tempted toward the bad fats anyway, making Laura's job even easier. And does she love her job! Through her vibration, she shares information with the rest of Ted that keeps him healthy and happy and moving forward on his true life path. Ted's cancer is gone, and the "real Ted" is now emerging.

Problems and Potentials of Pathway Care

Pathway healing is new to the world, and so it's difficult to offer statistics to evaluate it. This, then, is the major challenge in conducting pathway healing with confidence and care. It's a new process. It's an unknown. There aren't many pathway practitioners. It's hard to understand something that is new.

On the other hand, pathway practices are safe. The pathway system insists that you select healing methods that are tried and true and professionally recommended. Not only that, the pathway approach exponentially bolsters the effectiveness of traditional and alternative treatments. You can only get further ahead in the healing game by using the Four Pathways system.

Anecdotally, I have seen pathway therapies in and of themselves clear up problems and disorders, including cancer. This is because pathway processes are based in both scientific and spiritual truths. All energies do, in fact, reduce to three basic charges. All disease does boil down to a problem with information or vibration. Solve a problem at this elemental level, and you solve the problem.

In addition, there is a spiritual basis for all four pathways. We are made of flesh. As it clearly states in Genesis, the Bible of Islam, Judaism, and Christianity, from dust we were made; to dust we will return. Working the elemental pathway is about working with the core physical matter that composes us all. It is spiritual to address our very human concerns. All spiritualities emphasize the types of powers and forces available through the power pathway. Prophets, masters, gurus, and common people such as myself have accessed the supernatural to perform instant healing work in ourselves and others. The magic of the imagination pathway is a study of shamanism, a form of healing that cuts across all time periods and cultures. Certainly, there is a newly emerging scientific basis for the existence of antiworlds. The truth is, however, shamans have been walking these planes, performing their mysterious feats of magic, since time began. Finally, through the lens of the divine pathway we peer into the heart of heaven. Statistics are proving the power of prayer, faith, and belief. There is something greater than ourselves. There is a Greater Spirit, the Master Planner, the Diviner that created and sustains the Greater Reality. As we petition for help from above, we find that we are also petitioning to the part of the self that already knows his or her place in the Greater Reality. Our own spirit welcomes us into the arms of the Divine, glad that we are finally looking for what we truly need. Love.

Through the pathways, you are invited to find the real cause — and the ultimate need — that will bring your body back into balance. The answer exists, but isn't always available by looking through a microscope or taking an herb. Sometimes the only way to find the answer is to look into your own eyes.

chapter four

Chakras: Tools for Shifting

Between thumb and forefinger, Shepherd still pinched the fabric of reality.
"Do you feel the feel of it?" he asked.
"Feel what?"
"Feel how it works, the round and round of all that is."

— Clements, *Things Not Seen*[1]

Much of life is unseen. Can you see a flower before it pushes its way through the soil? Can you see the butterfly before it emerges from the cocoon? Can you see tomorrow before you reach it? True healing often requires a willingness to stretch into the unseen. Are you able to believe in what you can't touch? Use faith as a viewfinder for possibilities? Then you are ready to shift for healing.

Doorways Between Realities

I once stayed in a hotel called the Hotel Morocco with three other friends. As you could guess, we were in Morocco, at the far edge of the Sahara Desert and even farther away from vestiges of big-city luxuries. This village was so small that we were delighted to find that it even housed a hotel, and we were certainly not surprised to discover that we were the only guests encamped within.

We took a "suite," a conglomerate of rooms surrounding a central bathroom. There were only a couple of rooms on each of the six stories, and we occupied the majority of the second floor. We were happily ensconced in our extravagant setting — which we had obtained for a mere thirty dollars an evening — when one of us had to use the facilities.

The toilet wouldn't flush.

The caretaker grunted and provided us a key for a different room on the third floor, one that presumably had a functional toilet. We could remain in the suite and travel to a higher floor to use the rest room. That problem solved, we scoped out the transportation between floors. There were no stairwells — an anomaly that wouldn't have been allowed in America, but then again, we weren't in America. Rather, there was a glowing silver elevator, which appeared newer and better tended than any other apparatus in the hotel. So began the elevator trek to the toilet.

After laughing, we decided to freshen up for dinner. My friend Cathy was the first to decide to take a shower. Little surprise, but the shower in our personal suite didn't work. Via the elevator, we trudged back to the hotel lobby, where we were presented with yet another set of keys, this time for a working shower room on the fourth floor. After taking the elevator to the shower room, Cathy disappeared for a while, only to reappear in a fit of shivers. Yes, the shower worked — but the hot water didn't.

I hate cold showers, so quite willingly I visited our newfound friend, the hotel manager, who by this time probably wanted only to refund our thirty dollars and get rid of these troublesome tourists. Yes, there was hot water in the hotel, but we would have to find it. Armed with a set of key rings, we visited room after room, floor after floor, before figuring out that the water heated only on the first floor. The hardiest of us could continue to visit the shower on the fourth floor; as for me, I would indulge in the relative luxury of the tiny (hot) shower room on the first level.

The saga wasn't done. When it came time to brush teeth, we found out — can you imagine? — that our second-floor sink didn't work. For a working sink, we had to transport to the fifth floor.

For much of that night and into the next morning, one or the other of us was taking the elevator between floors. Sleeping on the second, hot showers on the first, the toilet on the third, and tooth brushing in the sink on the fifth. For the most part, we bypassed the third floor; Moroccan nights are cold, making a hot shower a seeming necessity. Thank goodness for the elevator.

The analogy may be a bit of a stretch, but your chakras are like the elevator running between the various levels of reality composing the infamous Hotel Morocco. The content material of your own four planes of existence, all of which create a larger and greater reality, might be more standardized — or at least a little less substandard — but the metaphor does work. Each chakra is a doorway, and all chakras are joined as if by an elevator shaft that allows you to shift from one place to another: from the elemental to the power pathway, the power to the imagination pathway; the imagination to the divine pathway; between any of the Four Pathways, in any order.

Understanding your chakras is critical to being a master self-healer. If you can use your chakras to shift from pathway to pathway, then you can also shift energies for healing. A simple breath on the divine pathway might be as powerful as a gust of wind on the elemental pathway. A spark of fire on the elemental pathway when conjoined with a power force can burn cancer right out of your body. These and other magical effects are the basis of shift healing and only possible for those who have learned to journey through their chakras.

Chakras in the Greater Reality

We all deal with the confounding truth that the invisible can be real. Your chakras might not show up on an X-ray film, but they are, nonetheless, quite real.

Is it so implausible, to believe in what you can't see? Our use of the Internet is entirely based on assuming the reality of the invisible. You can't see the information flowing through the Internet cyber body, yet after dialing in or, even more amazingly, tuning in through your wireless, you are plugged into this cyber realm, able to both upload and download data at will.

Within this cyber world, a chakra functions like a website. Your first chakra is its own particular site, composed with a specific set of data. Your second chakra is yet another site, featuring a different set of information. All of your chakras are linked together, making it easy for you to quickly tune into one after another. Through the cyber body that is the Internet, you can even transfer information from one site to the next, thus changing the content and character of each of these independent sites or chakras if you so desire.

The analogy gets more complicated if we tie in the fact that chakras exist on more than one pathway simultaneously. Imagine now that all of your chakras' websites are loaded on four independent servers, each of which emphasizes a different aspect of the programmed information. If pulling up a first-chakra site on server one, you'll see pictured the fundamental components of that chakra, including descriptions of its molecular, physically based structures. This would qualify as an elemental portrait of that chakra. On the power server, you find featured the supernatural energies creating that chakra. The imagination server presents your first chakra through mirror-like images that show you various magical ways to move energies from one world to another world, and the divine server offers the viewpoint of higher spiritual truths. Same chakra and same data, but different perspectives, all available to the energy expert who knows how to direct his or her consciousness in the same way that computer specialists know how to jump from website to website.

Most of us are unaware of the workings behind the Internet. Similarly, few of us know that our chakras, invisible organs of energy, are the powers fueling our bodies and our health. If we

Fear and the Four Pathways: Can Fear Help Make You Well?

One of the very real side effects of getting cancer is the terror of the diagnosis. Think of cancer, and you picture a balding head, wasted arms, and costly therapies. Contract cancer, and your heart grips in fear. Tell people that you have cancer, and they look away, crossing their hearts as if wishful thinking is a preventive measure.

Cancer is terrifying for several real reasons:

- We don't always know that we have it. *Cancer can be growing within us for ten to twenty years before it manifests itself in symptoms or reveals itself to diagnostic tools.*
- *We don't know for certain, in many cases, what really causes it.* There are a lot of theories and a lot of possible causes, but without definite answers it's hard to figure out what to do to keep from getting it.
- *We healers, no matter what our philosophy or method, don't always know how to make it go away.* Traditional treatments are invasive and make you sick. Alternative treatments are unpredictable, and they're so numerous, it's hard to sort them out.

Research isn't coming up with the answers.

All of these factors contribute to perhaps the greatest challenge: a feeling of helplessness. Cancer is caused by the out-of-control growth and spread of abnormal cells. And what feelings does cancer stimulate? Lack of control and the sense of being "abnormal." A cancer diagnosis seems like a death sentence because we don't know for sure that it won't kill us.

were healthy, we wouldn't need to know. Once cancer enters the picture, the self-healer is forced into a different position. Now it becomes important, maybe even imperative, to understand the functioning of these mystical energy bodies. By learning how to perceive and energetically work with your chakras, you can connect the two strongest variables of healing: information and vibration. You can apply the force of informed vibration to blast away your cancer or bolster your flagging immune system. You can also transfer energies between pathways, thereby benefiting from exponential change.

One of the key ideas in the Four Pathways philosophy is that fear can actually help make you well.

Okay, how can fear help?

On the pathways, your fear actually becomes a tool for directing the diagnosis and the healing. Ultimately, fear lies underneath every disease, including cancer. Fear is the opposite of love. All illnesses are, in the end, an attempt to find love to alleviate an internal sense of fear. We might fear that we aren't lovable. We might fear that we don't have enough power to accomplish our life purpose. We might fear that we don't deserve love, the good things in life, or life itself. We might fear that we aren't worthy of love from the Divine, other people, or even our own self. We might fear that we aren't a good person — that in fact we are evil or bad. Our core fear will be strongest in the part of the body, the aspect of the self, and the chakra and on the pathway that is holding the cause for your cancer. Find the fear, and you uncover the root of the cancer.

On the pathways, your whole self embraces your fearful self and provides the comfort and reassurance that you need to conduct a healing process. In pathway healing, you are taught how to follow your fear until finally you find the self who is living in fear. Talk with this self, embrace this self, get to know this self, and you discover the reasons for the cancer and the means that will heal it.

On the pathways, you ultimately are held in the arms of the real healer of fear and of cancer: the Divine. Your fearful self is already wrapped within the heart of the Divine. You have only to look into the eyes — and heart — of this self to discover that everything needed to completely heal and recover is already present. The Divine is within you, as you are also within the Divine.

You don't have to physically see your chakras for them to be real or for you to use them successfully, but you do have to know how to perceive them intuitively. These prisms of light are as real as the information in a website, and probably even more useful—you can transfer "viruses" out, not just in!

Spinning Wheels of Light

If you had attended school in ancient Egypt, you would have studied "chakra-ology." If you were one of the prize pupils among the ancient Maya, you would have called upon these innate powers to perform magic and healing. If you had been on the fast track to become a Siberian shaman, Hindu or Buddhist monk, Cherokee medicine person, or Chinese medical doctor, you would have been schooled in these points of wisdom.

There are twelve basic human chakras. Seven of them are body-based and emanate from your spine, where they spin in a vortex fashion, front and back.

Until recently, we had to take the word of the ancients and contemporary mystics that these energies exist, but science has caught up. Contemporary studies at learning institutions such as Duke University and University of California Los Angeles (UCLA) are proving the existence of chakras. Dr. Valerie Hunt of Stanford University, author of *The Science of Human Vibrations*, has produced striking documentation of the chakras. Healer Rosalyn Bruyere, in her book *Wheels of Light*, describes applications of Dr. Hunt's work. Bruyere and Hunt have actually created audiotapes of chakra sounds.[2]

Your chakras aren't magical. They are energy organs that work like your physical organs. Your liver transmutes blood; your pancreas alters hormones. Your heart and lungs convert weak blood into an oxygenated, life-giving substance. Chakras serve the same purpose: they transform energy from one form to another.

Chakras are often called "subtle energy bodies" because they vibrate at speeds and in spins that are difficult to perceive with the naked eye. Dr. Richard Gerber, author of *Vibrational Medicine*, asserts that "subtle energies at the etheric level are merely at a higher octave than the physical."[3] Chakras are as real as your liver or your heart, but their vibratory levels and functions are vaster and more expansive.

When their vibrations are seen psychically, each chakra is perceived as a different color. These colors connote the vibrational rate of that chakra. The red of the first chakra, for instance, describes the type of information-energy that runs through that energy center. The chakra isn't visually red; rather, red describes the energy spectrum controlled by that chakra. Red is the color of life, passion, and purpose.

Here are the primary locations of the chakras, their vibratory colors, and their overall missions. (My first book, *New Chakra Healing*, provides additional information.)

Chakra Basics

Chakra	Location	Color	Overall Mission
First	Genital area	Red	Security and survival
Second	Abdomen	Orange	Feelings and creativity
Third	Solar plexus	Yellow	Mentality and structure
Fourth	Heart	Green	Relationships and healing
Fifth	Throat	Blue	Communication and guidance
Sixth	Forehead	Purple	Vision and strategy
Seventh	Top of head	White	Purpose and spirituality
Eighth	Just above head	Black	Karma and universal linkages
Ninth	A foot above head	Gold	Soul programs and plans
Tenth	A foot below feet	Brown	Legacies and nature
Eleventh	A film around hands, feet,	Pink	Forces and energy conversion and body
Twelfth	Around the body and thirty-two points in the body	Clear	Ending of human self, access to the energy egg

The chakras have many functions in common, yet each chakra has independent and unique roles, as summarized in the table. The tasks of the chakras are informational and vibrational, the same root concepts we've been discussing in regard to energy. This means that chakras have the job of making energy work for you.

Chakras and Vibrational Information

Each of the twelve basic chakras regulates a set of physical, emotional, mental, and spiritual concerns, in addition to governing relational and psychic means of communicating. Fundamentally, chakras are communication organs of light. Like all organs, chakras rely upon information to function. In order to keep climbing the "chakra career ladder," chakras must be experts at communicating with information.

Communication always involves the same five basic steps, done in any order:

- Receiving information
- Decoding information
- Interpreting information
- Encoding a response
- Sending a response

Your physical organs perform these same tasks. They use chemicals, enzymes, DNA, and other materials to conduct their business. Chakras are also busy dealing with data, but with two astonishing variations. Your physical organs work only with sensory information; chakras handle not only sensory information but also psychic information. In fact, chakras can actually convert one speed of energy into the other, and vice versa!

Why can chakras do what your physical organs wouldn't even dare list on a job description? First, physical organs tend to vibrate within a limited frequency range. Chakras can work with the same frequencies as can their associated physical organs, but they can also perform octave shifts. This means that they can read or recognize information at the sensory level and the same information when it travels at the faster speed of the psychic level. As the chakras can process both "tones," they can easily translate a higher note to its lower pitch, and vice versa. Since a chakra can converse energetically on many levels, you can learn how to "read" a chakra for information, such as that causing disease or with the potential to heal disease. You can also vibrate various energies into a chakra and thus break physical organs free of maladies.

The second reason that chakras are so malleable is that they connect the Four Pathways. Chakras can bring information from one pathway to another. They can access a sacred spiritual idea on the divine pathway, usher it into the body on the elemental pathway, and then convert this star-studded idea into a mundane and practical means of delivering energy.

Chakras, as individual units, communicate using energies that match their unique vibrations. This means that while all chakras have certain basic information in common, such as the data that tells a chakra to be a chakra rather than a pancreas, each chakra is also responsible for processing very specific information.

Chakras subdivide the job of keeping you alive and healthy. Consider this table comparing the different organs managed by the different chakras.

Chakras in the Physical World

Chakra	Physiological Touchstones
One	Genital organs and endocrine system; coccygeal vertebrae; affects some adrenal, kidney, bladder, and excrement functions
Two	Intestines; part of the adrenal endocrine system; parts of kidney function; some aspects of reproductive system; sacral vertebrae and the neurotransmitters determining emotional responses to stimuli

Three	Pancreas endocrine system; all digestive organs in stomach area, including liver, spleen, gall bladder, stomach, and parts of kidney system; lumbar vertebrae
Four	Heart and lungs; circulatory and oxygenation systems; breasts; lumbar and thoracic vertebrae
Five	Thyroid endocrine gland; larynx, mouth, and auditory systems; lymph system; thoracic vertebrae
Six	Pituitary endocrine gland; parts of the hypothalamus; parts of the visual and olfactory systems (including the left eye); memory storage
Seven	Pineal endocrine gland; parts of hypothalamus, higher learning, and cognitive brain systems; parts of the immune system and brain glands affecting moods, emotions, and hormones
Eight	Thymus (immune system); memory retrieval functions; aspects of central nervous system (CNS); the right eye
Nine	Diaphragm; pineal gland; corpus callosum and other higher learning centers, including the cortex and neocortex
Ten	Feet, legs, and bones
Eleven	Skin and muscles
Twelve	Secondary chakric sites—there are at least thirty-two located throughout the body, including the knees, elbows, palms, and internal organs

Evaluating Cancer: The Role of Vibration

Stored within each chakra is all the data you've ever generated, accumulated, or created in regard to that chakra's areas of expertise. Because of the chakras' roles as record keepers, you can dig into your chakras to figure out the core cause of your cancer.

However, there are trillions upon trillions of bytes of information lurking inside of each chakra. Looking for the one fragment of data to explain your cancer is like searching for the proverbial needle in a haystack — especially when the needle can disguise itself to look like a piece of hay! There are probably countless potential causes for cancer in each chakra. Not all are activated; not all apply. Only a few master cancer cells do a tumor make. Only a select number of aneuploid cells establish the conditions for eventual malignancy.

If you're really going to heal from cancer, you must evaluate a chakra for vibration as well as information. Vibration produces an effect. When you vibrate the string of a violin, you hear a sound. You won't know if the violin is in tune or not until you make the strings vibrate. You won't make the A tone on a violin unless you draw the bow across the string or pluck the string with your finger. Vibration accounts for what actually occurs in your body in regard to health or disease. Vibration makes "reality" real.

Likewise, you can coexist for years or decades with cancerous conditions before developing cancer. Maybe your mother beat you when you were young. Perhaps you were exposed to chemical toxicity during childhood, or you smoked for years. None of this information will necessarily result in cancer, but any of it has potential to become the foundation for the disease. Data creates cancer or the conditions for cancer only when vibrated at a rate that breaks down the body's healthy systems and causes damage to healthy DNA.

Remember the theory about aneuploid cells? According to recent research, cancer might very well begin long before we see it in the body. Irregular cells exist in body tissue and become cancerous only when stimulated by powerful adversity. Bam! We're hit with a major trauma, and the vibrational intensity of this event overwhelms our system. The aneuploid cells succumb to the vibrational stress, and cancer develops.

A shocking short-term stress can also result in an immediate case of cancer. Intense exposure to radiation results in cancer within months, even days. For some people, intense exposure to a toxic person can have the same result.

Long-repressed feelings can build to a physical crisis. Long-term alcoholism eventually erodes the ability of our healthy cells to remain dutiful and strong. Whether information is transmitted physically, emotionally, mentally, or spiritually, it can all be translated into sensory information through a chakra.

This is why I use the idea of informed vibration when working the pathways for healing cancer.

Informed Vibration: The Basis of Chakra Healing

All vibration generates or is generated by information, and all information vibrates. Cancer is a vibrational as well as an informational disease. You can assess for information alone and get overwhelmed, or overlook the critical piece of data that is hiding underneath other data. You can work only vibrationally, and find yourself being impractical or, worse, creating harm. But looking for *informed vibration*—vibrations caused by or causing information critical to your case, and information vibrating in a way critical to your condition—greatly increases the chances for successful pathway healing. Working with informed vibration will accomplish the following through the chakras:

- Diagnose the primary causes of cancer
- Figure out potential cancer cures or treatments
- Shift informed vibration to heal cancer

When we're looking for informed vibration, we're looking for vibrating information that is doing or can do the following:

- Create the conditions for cancer
- Heal you from cancer

Consider that there is a pattern to cancer. In fact, there are six factors distinguishing cancer cells:

- Growth without normal "go" signals
- Growth despite "stop" commands
- Ability to hide from immune helpers
- Ability to co-opt nearby blood vessels
- Near immortality
- Ability to spread

From somewhere, cancer cells are getting the message to grow, even though they are abnormal. They can't or won't read the data that says to stop growing. They emanate information cloaking them with invisibility and another set of commands that convinces the body to provide their needs. Healthy cells can divide only seventy times. Cancer cells run data that coerces the DNA to keep on going, much as if hooked up to an eternal battery. And they emit communication that destroys the circuitry keeping them locked into a specific body site.

You can attempt to work only with information telling the cancer to grow, but this will tell you only half the story. Let's say that your cancer began when you were exposed to lead paint as a child. Lead paint can be understood as a chemical equation. It's not the information in this equation that causes the cancer. You didn't swallow a piece of paper with numbers and elements written on it! It's the *vibration* of this information that creates a cancer.

But it's not enough to know the cancer is caused by lead paint. A good investigative mind can tell you that. *Knowing the cause does not make a cancer disappear.*

Unfortunately, I meet a lot of people who believe that just figuring out the core root of a cancer can heal the cancer. In the holistic field, for instance, some practitioners give affirmations—positive thoughts to help their cancer clients achieve an optimistic attitude and therefore increase the immune system's strength.

An affirmation, such as "I am healing from cancer," is meaningless if your body can't vibrationally receive the message, or if the mes-

sage itself doesn't hold a vibrational impact for your body. The impact is created by the ability of your body to "read" and use the vibration of that message. A weak, half-uttered fluttering of the phrase is going to slide right over those cancer cells, which might just say, "Thanks for the breeze."

I also meet a lot of people who think it's enough to work just vibrationally. We've all experienced the immediate benefits of vibrational healing. Ever listened to a lovely symphony when stressed? Through the vibration, carrying messages you receive as "peaceful," you become more serene. This data is actually communicated into your fifth chakra, which is located in your throat. If the intensity is powerful enough, the fifth chakra is able to amplify the meaning of the music or vibration and enable the rest of your body to conform to the soothing tones.

Many physicians are now using vibration for healing and diagnosis. About thirty years ago, scientists began observing that NASA astronauts developed something they called *space sickness*. Determining that the cause was the decreased exposure to the earth's magnetism, space shuttles were then equipped with magnetic-field generators.

Researchers have established parameters to figure out healthy or unhealthy amounts of magnetics. Tumors grow faster in a 60-Hz magnetic field. Yet lower magnetic doses seem to increase the delivery of oxygen to the body's tissues. Color, sound, and symbol therapy—all instruments that deliver vibration—have made phenomenal differences in people's health and well-being.

Yet it's not enough to just vibrate any bit of information. For instance, I could insist that I'm only going to play one of the four strings on a violin, and that's it. I like the A string and only that string. What happens if I need to hit a low C, a note that you can't generate from the A string? As much as I might vibrate it, the A string will not produce a low C.

Most people use some variety of traditional medicine when treating cancer. Radiation, for instance, is actually a form of vibrational healing. Physicians hope that the toxic energy waves will break the cancer's rhythm. Unable to continue its pattern, the cancer should then die.

The problem is, you have very little idea what information you're carrying into your body on these radioactive waves. Are these waves informationally programmed by a lab technician? Then they are possibly resonant with data about the scrambled eggs that he ate for breakfast. This incoming information might make you hungry, but it won't go far in curing your cancer. Perhaps the radiation is neutral. Neutrality produces no effect. That's not bad, but that's not good enough to eliminate your cancer. Perhaps the radiation picks up on your own programming. Like attracts like. Radioactivity runs at certain frequencies, and will absorb concepts and feelings that match its vibratory levels. My guess is that these concepts will more likely focus on doubts and fears than on hopes and dreams.

Is it really different if you work holistically? Some holistic practitioners use light-based therapy to address cancer. The idea is to support the body with vibrations that support life and wellness. Does anyone ever ask what information is loaded into these streams of light? Whose messages are carried on those particle streams? Scrambled eggs for breakfast again? Let's say that you don't really want to get well, or that you are scared of your doctor. These pieces of data can flow right into the supposedly healing light *and further indoctrinate your body*. You have now created more harm than good.

The bottom line is that you must work with both information and vibration together to heal cancer.

Searching for Harmful Vibrational Information

Cancer cells are vibrationally "out of tune" with the vibrations of your healthy cells. They have lost their capacity to hold your body's natural rhythms. Cancer cells are in discord with your inherent spiritual harmonies: they are vibration information that is bad for you.

There are really only three types of information communicated via the chakras. There is *useful information*, which assists and sustains you in meeting your life purpose. This data supports health. There is *neutral information*, which doesn't do much of anything. It doesn't hurt you, nor does it serve you. Then there's *harmful information*, which is detrimental to achieving your spiritual mission and can actually create disease and lack of health. When searching for cancer causes, you only want to distinguish useful and neutral information from harmful information vibrating against your basic harmonic. You're looking for bad programs that have been activated.

Innately, a chakra runs on programming determined by your inner spirit. *Programming* is your spirit's master code, which directs the chakras to select information telling you what to do, how to feel, and what to think. You are a spiritual being, and your spiritual perfection is programmed right into every chakra, every cell, and every aspect of your being. You are already whole, and buried within your chakras is the programming for wholeness in health and well-being. You just don't remember that you already remember wholeness!

If chakras were simply allowed to hum along without interference, your body would be healthy and you'd be happy all the time. You'd work only with useful information and ignore or discard all else. Fortunately or unfortunately, chakras are affected by life experience. As communication organs, they can record information that leads to learning, wisdom, love, and well-being. They can just as easily store data that causes bad beliefs, judgments, and disease.

Some of the data that you've recorded is bad for you, plain and simple. In computer language, your hard drive is fine, your first software was great and loaded correctly, but you have acquired a computer virus — a bad program that interferes with your software and keeps you from accessing all your capabilities. If you have cancer, then you're running a program that is making you sick. You're making decisions, consciously or unconsciously, based on bad programming.

Bad programs distort the natural vibratory rates of your chakras and can cause physical, emotional, mental, spiritual, relational, and psychic malfunctions. One or all of these types of malfunctions can result in cancer.

There are several types of bad programs, which I call *strongholds*. A stronghold occurs when beliefs or feelings are permanently paired with each other in a harmful manner.

Constantly, beliefs and feelings join to forge *emotions: "emotion" is a great way to move "e-nergy" into "motion."* You need emotions. If you see a fire in the pantry and panic, the energy produced by the emotion can get you to run out the door and save your life. But if you continue to partner the thought of "fire is dangerous" with the feeling of panic, you've created an emotional stronghold. You'll flee when someone so much as strikes a match in your presence. An *emotional stronghold* is therefore a harmful pairing of a belief and a feeling, occurring when these energies stay locked together even after they don't need to be.

You can also pair a belief with a belief and produce a disastrous response. This is the basis of a *mental stronghold.* For instance, you might think that ice cream is highly nutritious because your grandfather told you so. Then you learn that it's good to eat lots of nutritious foods. What happens if you keep these two ideas married? Ice cream itself is neither good nor bad, but the effect it produces — obesity — when eaten too much is unhealthy.

Strongholds create patterns, and these can be partially responsible for the conditions underlying certain types of cancer. A *pattern* is a response stuck to a stimulus, in which you keep acting the same way continuously, even though circumstances have changed. Because of a mental or emotional stronghold, you might develop the pattern of smoking every time you are stressed. Smoking is one of the leading causes of cancer. This kind of pattern can kill you.

When working the pathways, you must sort the harmful data from the helpful or neutral. This is the key to figuring out your diagnosis, which is the basis of working the pathways correctly. You have to match the treatment with the diagnosis. After all, you wouldn't try and heal a cold the same way you'd deal with hunger pains, would you? A muffin won't assuage many sniffles. Of course, in pathway healing, you can conceivably program a muffin to heal your cold. Just as chemotherapy chemicals can be programmed with information to build the body's immune system — processes described in chapters 6 and 7 — so can you alter the purpose of a muffin!

On the elemental pathway, the causes of cancer number in the thousands — from poor diet, to smoking, to repressed feelings, to nasty relationships. On the power pathway, we're dealing with forces, which support the existence or elimination of cancers and cancer-causing agents. In this context, I am referencing forces that are supernaturally appearing energies that can be directed to create change. On the imagination pathway, you're basically dealing with the choice of cancer versus the choices available on other worlds. On the divine pathway perspective, cancer isn't a problem. It's a doorway into love.

How can you sort through all these details to find an informed vibration that can help you see into every pathway?

You look for the basics.

Diagnosis and Healing: The Basics of Informed Vibration

Making the right fundamental diagnosis will help you decide which information-energies to use in healing from cancer and which pathways to use. It will also enable you to transfer energies between pathways. You don't have to look any further than back to the basics of energy.

Again, all cancers are based on negative, positive, or neutral energies, or a mixture of some or all of these. A negative-based cancer is going to create more depression than other types and will involve patterns of emotional strongholds. A positive-based cancer reflects anxiety and patterns involving mental strongholds. Neutral-based cancers usually revolve around a core misperception. Knowing the precise mixture of your cancer will tell you how to choose treatment on the elemental pathway; select forces on the power pathway; make energy exchange ideas on the imagination pathway; and open to the Divine on the divine pathway. Here is a chart to help you figure out what these various types of cancer energies might "look" like psychically (in your mind's eye). I have included a description of cancer coloration, which is the color that these various cancers appear to me. You might feel overwhelmed at the thought of working energetically if you aren't used to it or feel underprepared for the task. As simple as it sounds, the key is to trust your intuition. It will show you truth. Toward this end, you will learn more about tapping into your innate intuition in chapter 5.

Positive-Based Cancers

- Coloration when cancerous: yellow or a discolored yellow, or an off white.
- Cancer will psychically appear as swirling or spinning areas of yellow or yellow-white energy; if you analyze the information in these areas, you can determine the nature of the spiritual misperception creating the discord.
- If psychically examining the DNA, you will see yellow or yellow-white energies erasing the needed genes.
- Coloration when healing or healthy: gold, or sometimes white.
- Patient is anxious, scared, can't settle down.
- Affected chakras spin too fast and clockwise.
- In general, positive-based illnesses will originate in the

second, fourth, sixth, eighth, tenth, and twelfth chakras, although this is not a hard-and-fast rule, as cancer is a tricky and unpredictable disease.

- Positive cancers will create or be caused by an alkaline imbalance.
- Elementally, there are usually too much water and other yeast-, fungal-, or bacterial-producing elements in the body.
- Managing energy bodies — the energy organs of the elemental pathway — are disconnected from each other.
- Feelings are fear-based and cause anxieties and worry about the future.
- The patient's issues will reflect fears about the future.
- Auric field is too thin.
- Coloration of affected chakras is too light.
- Tones of affected chakras are too high.
- Symbols will tend to be circular, but will be broken or misshapen, or energetically connect the cancer patient to bad sources.
- The number indicating the cancer will be odd rather than even, as this person will essentially have difficulties placing power within the self or defining his or her personal role in the universe. Hence, the adopted and mistaken spiritual beliefs are oriented toward using love to avoid personal power.
- *Main issue to uncover: spiritual. Must provide new data to change the vibratory rate into the correct harmonic.*

Negative-Based Cancers

- Coloration when cancerous: blue; the most critical cancers are cobalt or deep blue.
- Cancer will psychically look like deadened or dull blobs of bluish material; if you assess the information within, you will uncover psychic or physical toxins; repressed feelings

or parts of the self; and cords and other dynamics, such as interference.

- If psychically examining the DNA, you will spot blue or dark energies creating tight structures that keep the genes from fully activating or flowing properly.
- Coloration when healing or healthy: black.
- The patient is depressed, despairing, stuck in the past.
- Affected chakras spin too slowly or counterclockwise.
- The chakras bearing negative-based illnesses are usually the first, third, fifth, seventh, ninth, and eleventh, though this isn't a strict rule with cancer, which is highly unpredictable.
- Negative cancers will create or be caused by an acidic imbalance.
- Elementally, there is usually too much of fire and other viral-inciting elements in the body.
- Managing energy bodies on the elemental pathway are too connected with each other; there is a lack of independent functioning.
- Feelings are depressed, causing sadness and rage; feelings may not be one's own, but probably at least partially sublimated from others.
- Patient's issues are rooted in the past; there is a lack of release from prior situations.
- Auric field is often too thick or murky.
- Coloration of the affected chakras is dark, heavy, and blobby.
- Tones of the affected chakras are too low.
- Symbols will tend to be boxy, but will be too thick, broken, misshapen, or misused. They will indicate cords or other energetic connections to interference.
- Numbers indicating the cancer will be in even sequence, like 2, 4, 6, 8, 10, or 12, reflecting associations with unhealthy energies and interference. The issues actually

reflect misunderstandings about love, which damage numbers that concern issues about love.

- *Main issue to uncover: power. Must vibrate the energies so as to access information that can be used for personal empowerment.*

Neutron-Based Cancers

- Coloration when cancerous: red or a discoloration of red, such as muddy, brick red.
- Cancer will psychically look like red material standing out on a flat plane. The only "life" in this person is the cancer. All life energy flows into the cancer, and you might see cordage, such as life-energy cords, going into the cancerous area.
- If psychically examining the DNA, you will spot red, inflamed energies drawing the life force out of the cellular structure.
- Coloration when healing or healthy: pink.
- Patient is apathetic, nonnurturing, confused.
- Affected chakras don't spin, or they move very little.
- Any chakra can be affected.
- Misinformed neutrons create both acidic and alkaline imbalances in various parts of the body.
- Elementally, there is almost always too much metal present (to serve as protection).
- Feelings are nonexistent or hard to discern.
- The cancer has few or no connections to anything, anyone, or any time period. This situation reflects the patient's tendency to be unable to move forward or backward in life, in at least one major life area, like health, relationships, or work.
- Auric fields lack intensity and fluidity; they are stuck in one position.
- Colorations of affected chakras will be bland, though consistent, except for the area showing the cancer, which will be red.

- Tonality of affected chakras will be flat and lack pitch and depth.
- Symbols will be of one variety and extremely fixated. They will not move or flow.
- The system will not have a variety of numbers; everything will be the same.
- *Main issue to uncover: address love and power issues. The first is love of life; there are reasons that this person is frightened of love, life, or both. The second is fear of personal power; the ill person fails to perceive the extent of personal power available for making life changes. Essentially, the patient needs to learn how to vibrate with life energy so as to give and receive love.*

Working the Chakras at the Source

One of the most confusing aspects of working with cancer compared with working with other diseases is that cancer can involve a mix of energetics. Some cancers are negative, others partially negative, and others neutral. You'll gain your greatest success by keeping the process simple. I'll explain how.

Healing on the pathways involves working energetically from the primary source of a cancer. In general, you want to begin and end all chakric cancer work at the cancer's primary site. To do this, you have only to figure out the primary chakra site for the cancer. From here, you can figure out the reason the cells went awry and access the pathway that can best provide healing.

It's not as difficult as you might think to source a cancer. Armed with the knowledge of the particular part of the body regulated by each chakra, you can identify the chakra in closest proximity to the cancer, then pinpoint the chakric doorway into the Greater Reality.

The following chart shows you which chakras are most frequently associated with which cancers. For more insights, refer also to the table of physiological chakra touchstones earlier in this chapter.

Chakras and Affiliated Cancers

First Chakra	Second Chakra	Third Chakra	Fourth Chakra
Vaginal Skin (also eleventh chakra) Rectal Prostate (also second chakra) Testicular Cervical Adrenal	Colon Prostate (also first chakra) Ovarian Uterine Kidney (also third chakra) Bladder	Stomach Liver Pancreatic Gall bladder Spleen (such as in Hodgkin's disease; also fifth chakra) Esophageal (also fourth) Adrenal Kidneys (always second chakra, sometimes also third chakra)	Lung Breast Heart Esophageal (also third chakra) Leukemia (also tenth chakra)

Fifth Chakra	Sixth Chakra	Seventh Chakra	Eighth Chakra
Thyroid Larnyx Oral Lymphatic Tracheal Hodgkin's disease (also third chakra) Non-Hodgkin's lymphoma	Pituitary Eye (left eye)	Pineal (also ninth chakra) Hypothalamus Brain, including those cancers affecting higher learning centers (also ninth chakra) Cancers caused originally by depression of immune system	Thymus Some types of central nervous system cancers Eye (right eye) Cancers carried over from past lives or caused by sorcery

Ninth Chakra	Tenth Chakra	Eleventh Chakra	Twelfth Chakra
Diaphragm Pineal (also seventh chakra) Brain, including those affecting higher learning cancers (also seventh chakra) Cancers taken on to "help the world," such as those absorbed from a radiation fallout	Bone Cancers caused by the environment, such as in environmental poisoning Genetically based cancers Cancers created from familial or ancestral interference or bindings Many childhood cancers	Skin (also first chakra)	Cancers affecting secondary sites, including joints

On Associated Cancers

Chakras often store the energies creating cancer exactly in or on the organs associated with that chakra. For instance, lung cancer is a fourth-chakra cancer. The lungs are one of the primary physical organs composing the fourth chakra; therefore, it is easy to link this type of cancer with the fourth chakra. What about bone cancer in the shoulder joint, however? Sometimes the body creates cancer in a physical location that is "off site" of a primary organ, in order to preserve the organ from harm. Heart issues are often stored in the shoulders, for instance, so that the body can maintain the integrity of the heart muscle. Therefore, shoulder cancer might reflect issues involving both the fourth chakra and perhaps the twelfth chakra, which regulates joints. A malignant tumor near the left eye probably involves the sixth chakra; one near the right eye might stem from eighth chakra issues.

Informed Vibration in Action

Consider what might happen to someone who represses anger for forty years.

Anger is information that vibrates at a certain rate. If we don't let it out of the body, it will get stored in a part of the body that matches it vibrationally. This process involves hundreds of chemical, biological, and hormonal reactions. For the sake of understanding the energetics of an anger-based cancer, we'll look mainly at the role of vibration and information through an example, although I will provide a cursory look at a few of the chemicals involved in anger-based cancer. Our lead character is Maria, who fell prey to ovarian cancer. Let's look at her story.

The information of the anger energy contains a message — to establish boundaries — but Maria doesn't do that. She'd rather believe that anger is dangerous. Vibrationally, we're looking at a situation in which anger has superseded the innate, positive programming that once kept Maria's ovaries happy and healthy. The energetic outcome is a negative, reverse spiral pattern in her second chakra. The longer Maria represses her anger, the more intense the pattern. More anger leads to more problems, as the vibratory rate of this anger begins to distort all "nonanger" vibrations in the ovaries.

Anger is an inflammatory energy, not only psychically but also in terms of the body. Anger involves a particular sequencing of peptides produced by the hypothalamus as well as other glands and organs. Maria's anger produces neuropeptides that fill cellular receptors in her body. Where her internal programming allows, the cells clear the anger-neuropeptides when she is done being angry. However, the programming in her second chakra and in particular in her ovaries doesn't allow her to release the anchored neuropeptides. Eventually the physical frequencies of Maria's anger, now stuck in her ovaries, build to the point of inflammation and infection.

The infection intensifies until her body forms a cyst around it. Cysts are protective encasings for energies that are dangerous to the body. Perhaps the cyst forms in Maria's right ovary, although both ovaries are full of anger. The right side of the body tends to relate to issues with men, power, or our own masculine nature. The left side of the body commonly references issues with women, love, or our own feminine nature. If, for instance, Maria began repressing anger in reaction to her father's misuse of anger, her right ovary would be more affected than her left.

Now the anger is physically stuck. Unable to dissipate, it continues to rage until Maria's pH balance and balance of elements (air, wood, water, and other basic natural properties) are in complete disarray. The vibratory rate of this anger-infection doesn't match the innate, healthy vibration of the right ovary. The anger vibration eventually distorts the information carried within vulnerable, sensitive cells, which now mutate, forming the basis for cancer. Seen biochemically, the neuropeptides locked into the cellular receptors eventually emit chemicals that infiltrate into the center of the cells. These invasive chemicals can eventually erode the core DNA program, causing cancer.

While this is occurring on the elemental pathway, Maria's other pathways are responding in kind. On the power pathway, the spiritual energetic forces respond to Maria's repression of anger. They may attach a generative spiritual force to the anger to keep it riled up. They may attach a degenerative spiritual force to the healthy cells to keep them weak.

The imagination pathway makes sure other realities don't impose on the one with cancer. On the divine pathway, Maria's higher self smiles. Maybe at some point Maria will learn the lesson of the first channel of light, the higher aspect of the first chakra. This is an important lesson in self-care; she deserves to take care of herself. If Maria could learn to express her anger, she would be more self-loving. The divine pathway self awaits insight.

All the pathways work together, not only to reinforce an illness, but to heal you of the patterns creating an illness. *Through your chakras, you can actually change a quantum of possibility into an atom of reality.* It's just a matter of learning how. Let's say, for instance, that Maria comes to realize that anger plays an important role in self-love, the learning of the divine pathway. Upon her accepting the necessity of using anger energy to establish healthy personal boundaries, the stuck anger-neuropeptides would begin releasing from her ovaries. The initial physical cause of the inflammation and infection would alter the chemical composition of the cancer site, perhaps allowing elemental healing methods such as chemotherapy, positive self-talk, or diet to flush the cancer cells. Over time, her "change of mind" would establish new neurological patterns within her entire system, and she would respond differently under stress. When feeling violated, Maria's brain might not even respond with anger at all. Perhaps divine pathway ideals like faith or hope or understanding would take over instead, positive energies that, when they flood the body, actually bolster the immune system. By understanding the importance of the healthy use of anger, Maria's entire body would alter its biochemistry and promote healing instead of disease. As your body can, as well.

chapter five

Intuition: Tools for Energy Mapping

In the midst of all the din and the flurry, he had suddenly had a strange feeling stronger than any he had ever known; he had been aware that someone was trying to tell him something, something that had missed him because he could not understand the words. Not words exactly; it had been like a kind of silent shout. But he had not been able to pick up the message, because he had not known how.

— Susan Cooper, *The Dark Is Rising*[1]

The most important tool you need for healing is already within you. It is your intuition. You've been using your intuition your entire life, but may not have yet grasped the full brilliance and facility of this gift. In its evolved state, your intuition can help you diagnose and heal. It is your main mechanism for planning and prayer. It is your connection to all parts of yourself and the Divine. Connect with your intuition, and you connect to yourself.

The Basics of Shift Healing: Using Your Intuition

In order to diagnose and heal through your chakras, you must use your psychic abilities in the form of intuition. With your intuition, you not only diagnose and perform healing, but you can also energy map and shift between pathways.

In this chapter, I'm going to briefly describe intuition: what it is, why you have it, and what it does for you. You'll take the Psychic Style Quiz, so you can figure out which innate gifts would be best to use intuitively for healing. Then I'm going to show you how to use your intuition to energy map — to sketch or sense maps of energy that will help you use the chakras to work the Four Pathways program. Finally, I'm going to help you identify which of the Four Pathways you might want to work for a particular concern. You'll then be ready to play on any of the pathways easily and effectively.

This chapter includes a special insert about energy information and tools you'll need for energy map healing. You can reference this insert for terms when energy mapping.

The Intuitive Edge: Learning What You Know How to Do

Accessing your innate psychic abilities enables you to hone them into surgical equipment far more precise than any in a medical operating room. Your intuition can enable you to pinpoint the source of a cancer, determine its type, identify the best technique for healing, and shift energies between pathways.

Intuition is applied psychism. Everyone is psychic. The psychic ability is simply the process of communicating with fast-moving information-energy. Remember, information can move faster than the speed of light. When traveling this fast, psychic energy breaks the spacetime barrier. You can know about an event before it happens, determine the nature of energy in a room you've never been in before, or discover who's on the phone before you answer.

Each chakra houses a particular psychic ability. Some of our chakric gifts are more strongly developed than others, because some abilities are more important to your spiritual destiny than others. I have always wanted to be a writer, so my fifth chakra's basic psychic attribute was fairly well honed even when I was a child. The gifting in this area is called verbal sympathy, and it relates to hearing words, messages, sounds, and music from all planes and dimensions. When I was a small child, I would often lie in bed listening to the ghosts in my house, hearing angels sing in the wind, and tuning into the thoughts of my parents. You, too, have gifts unique and special to you.

The basic psychic capabilities are instinctive and ensure our survival. Though they are inherent to us all, most adults aren't in touch with their psychic qualities. This usually occurs during childhood because of lack of support or because of fear. We might have shared our psychic insights when growing up, only to be told to knock it off, that we were stupid, or that we were doing something bad. Society tends to fear something that is powerful and that can potentially empower the person rather than the whole group. Until recently there has been little support to help individuals develop their psychic gifts. These gifts are key to your own healing process, and you'll need to tap into them for pathway healing.

Using Your Intuition

Using your psychic talents is not something you should just rush off and begin doing. The psychic world is fraught with dangers and misperceptions. It's not easy to discover what the various psychic signs really mean, or to distinguish a harmful from a helpful source, or an applicable message from a nonapplicable one. It takes a lot of time and practice.

Psychic abilities are the raw, base skills of communicating with psychic energy. Programming from the following sources can affect psychic abilities positively or negatively:

- Childhood experiences
- Parents and extended family
- Ancestral beliefs and traditions
- Peers
- Schools
- Religious institutions
- The media
- Your community
- The culture at large
- Your soul and spirit
- The Divine
- The world of spirits

The vulnerability of psychic abilities to interference may be one of the main reasons that so many people are scared of these talents. But your psychic gift is too great a tool to ignore, however, as it is really the only nonmechanical way to gather information and work vibrationally. Best of all, the power to tap into psychic information lies within you!

Intuition Involves Boundaries

Intuition is psychic ability used with boundaries and parameters for safety. As used in psychology, the term *boundaries* refers to our response to the need to be safe. An example of a sensory boundary is a fence. A fence around your yard can keep out strangers and keep in your kids. Psychic boundaries are just as important as sensory boundaries. You might say that psychic boundaries are the fences that prescribe your level of emotional, mental, spiritual, and physical security.

Why are psychic boundaries so important? If the doorbell rings, would you open the door without checking out who is there? Especially if there has been a serial killer in the neighborhood? No — a smart person wants to be safe and checks first.

Psychic parameters are guidelines set to screen information and to keep your vibration attuned with your harmonic. A parameter is like a stop sign. It insists that information sources must stop before entering your energy field. You can then decide whether to admit them or not.

Regarding the pathways, a trained psychic ability or intuitive faculty can enable you to move energy from place to place, bring energies where needed, and release energies causing problems. It enables you to tap into sources from the eight major levels of psychic sources:

1. The physical world, including animals, plants, elements, and spirits of nature
2. The emotional plane, including feelings and emotions from other people and entities
3. The mental plane, including thoughts, beliefs, ideas, and fears from other people and entities
4. The relational plane, including anything or anyone, alive or dead, to whom you have a bond or connection
5. The energetic plane — the world in which all energy interacts, also containing the beings that attend these processes
6. The soul plane, which involves all communication between your soul and those of others
7. The world of spirits, which includes all spirits, alive or dead, positive or negative
8. The world of the spirit, the base of which is the Divine

There are certain sources that are more helpful and available on one pathway than on another. Use your intuition to access these, making sure you have established solid boundaries and parameters regarding what is acceptable or not. Several types of invisible sources are described in the insert of this chapter, and I will highlight certain sources for each pathway in the individual chapters for each of the pathways. As you further use your intuition and progress on the pathways, you will find that your gifts develop further, as do your connections into the spiritual worlds.

Sympathy Versus Empathy

The main difference between psychic abilities and intuitive abilities is the use of *sympathy* versus *empathy*.

Sympathizers often take on external energies, literally absorbing them through the skin and into their bodies. Many cancers are partially caused by this practice. Your body cannot process energy that is unlike its own. Others' energies disrupt the information and vibration of your own system and can lead to cancerous mutations. You should sympathize only when you know exactly what the incoming energy is going to do, and you are sure it will revive your own harmonic, such as when undergoing the process of transmission. *Transmission* is the full transference of energy from being to being. It is often employed by masters or gurus and is used frequently on the divine pathway.

Empathy involves registering energy rather than assuming it. A physical sympathizer, for instance, can potentially take another's cancer right into his or her own body. I had a client named Clara who did this. Both Clara and her mother had breast cancer: her mother contracted it first. As soon as Clara figured out that she was absorbing her mother's breast cancer, she decided to put up better psychic boundaries. After imaging white light protection around her energy system, Clara mentally released the cancer energy. Rather than inserting it back into her mother's body, she returned it to her mother's higher self.

When working with absorbed energies, it's important to hand them to another's higher self, spirit, or spiritual guidance, or directly to the Divine, as you don't want to be responsible for causing someone else more problems than they already have. If at a subconscious level you've "agreed" to take care of someone else's energy, you are partially responsible for your own predicament, but you are not responsible for correcting another's situation or for supporting them in their disease process.

By establishing proper psychic boundaries and refusing to caretake (or take care of) her mother's issues, Clara released herself from the cancer process. She thus transformed from being a physical sympathizer to a physical empathizer. A physical empathizer can read or perceive data through his or her first chakra, but doesn't take this energy inside of the self.

The Psychic Style Quiz

What are your most appropriate and keen intuitive gifts to use for energy mapping? This quick quiz will give you a start on figuring out this answer; a more detailed test is available in *Advanced Chakra Healing: Energy Mapping.*

Respond to the following questions by selecting the most applicable number. A "zero" indicates you've never experienced this phenomenon; a "five" indicates that you experience the phenomenon constantly.

1. I sense others' physical conditions in my own body.

   0 1 2 3 4 5

2. When I'm at the movies or reading a book, I feel the characters' experiences in my own body.

   0 1 2 3 4 5

3. I always know what others are feeling emotionally.

   0 1 2 3 4 5

4. I am like a human sponge for others' emotions.

   0 1 2 3 4 5

5. I often know information I've never been taught.

   0 1 2 3 4 5

6. I sense, in my stomach, whether or not someone is being honest.

0 1 2 3 4 5

7. I easily predict the outcome of people's relationships.

0 1 2 3 4 5

8. I often find myself helping people with their relationship concerns.

0 1 2 3 4 5

9. Words will come to me as soon as I open my mouth.

0 1 2 3 4 5

10. I can hear words, tones, or guidance from beings that aren't present.

0 1 2 3 4 5

11. I often get information via pictures in my mind.

0 1 2 3 4 5

12. I get visions that tell me what to do.

0 1 2 3 4 5

13. It's easy for me to sense right from wrong.

0 1 2 3 4 5

14. I sense what the Divine plans are for myself or other people.

0 1 2 3 4 5

15. I have always been able to enter a trance state and connect with different worlds.

0 1 2 3 4 5

16. I remember having been alive before, and I can sometimes see others' past lives.

0 1 2 3 4 5

17. I am naturally concerned about the global impact that actions may have.

0 1 2 3 4 5

18. I seem to know what's going on in others' souls.

0 1 2 3 4 5

19. I know myself as one with nature.

0 1 2 3 4 5

20. I get my guidance and energy from the natural world.

0 1 2 3 4 5

21. I can command energies and forces to do my will.

0 1 2 3 4 5

22. Through my hands and feet, I can move energy at my own bidding.

0 1 2 3 4 5

Scoring, Part I: Add your scores for the following pairs of answers:

Questions 1 and 2
Questions 3 and4
Questions 5 and 6
Questions 7 and 8
Questions 9 and 10
Questions 11 and 12
Questions 13 and 14
Questions 15 and 16
Questions 17 and 18
Questions 19 and 20
Questions 21 and 22

How many tens do you have? How many zeros? These numbers could indicate strong or weak tendencies in each of the eleven major psychic styles, according to these divisions:

Questions 1 and 2	Chakra One, Physical
Questions 3 and 4	Chakra Two, Feeling
Questions 5 and 6	Chakra Three, Mental
Questions 7 and 8	Chakra Four, Relational

Questions 9 and 10	Chakra Five, Verbal
Questions 11 and 12	Chakra Six, Visual
Questions 13 and 14	Chakra Seven, Spiritual
Questions 15 and 16	Chakra Eight, Shadow
Questions 17 and 18	Chakra Nine, Soul
Questions 19 and 20	Chakra Ten, Natural
Questions 21 and 22	Chakra Eleven, Force

Scoring, Part II: List your chakras and their corresponding gifts in order from strongest to weakest. Now read "Chakra Psychic Gifts" to determine how you might best use your strongest gifts for intuitive energy mapping.

Chakra Psychic Gifts

Here is an overview of the types of gifts innate to each chakra. I have explained each psychic gift, then added advice on how to use this inherent gift in an intuitive fashion. Additionally, I have offered a few words regarding the application of each gift in energy mapping and healing cancer.

Chakra One: Physical sympathy. You are very physical and naturally know what is occurring in your own or others' bodies. You can tend, however, to absorb others' illnesses and make them your own. If you have cancer, determine if someone else's energies are the cause of your disrupted cellular functions. Tied with this tendency is the ability to perform *psychometry*: reading the information stored within physical objects. You can use this skill to see if an herb, supplement, or treatment modality is correct for your body. You will sense answers in your body in response to questions; trust these physical sensations. Something helpful will "feel good" and make you "feel better"; a poor choice will "feel bad" and make you "feel worse."

Chakra Two: Feeling sympathy. Feeling-oriented, you easily take on others' feelings. Figure out if any aspect of the cancer is caused from others' feelings or your vibrational sensitivity to them. There are feeling energies in almost all vibrations, including those on the power pathway. Use your sensitivity to read feeling energies. Which should you take in? Which should you deflect? Your feelings will tell you which energies are healthy and can heal you. Positive energies will make you feel lighter and happier; those you sense you should reject or release will cause depression or anxiety.

Chakra Three: Mental sympathy. You input psychic information constantly and can organize it logically. When working energetically, trust what you simply perceive or know. You are *clairsentient* — clear sensing — which means you obtain accurate perceptions about information from any or all of the pathways. You'll be highly skilled at assessing beliefs and patterns in working with cancer.

Chakra Four: Relational sympathy. You are highly sensitive to relationship concerns. Your most precise way of working intuitively is to figure out the relationship between cancer and other factors, including various aspects of yourself, external variables, outside energies, and the Divine. Simply open the back side of your heart chakra to bring through Divine love, and you can channel healing energies from near and far. Ask always for wisdom from the "High Heart" — the part of you connected to the Divine — and you can trust your diagnostic and energetic healing skills.

Chakra Five: Verbal sympathy. You receive psychic data as tones or verbal or written messages. This gift, called *clairaudience,* means clear hearing. Confirm you are sourcing helpful energies or entities by setting clear parameters and boundaries or by calling on a gatekeeper — an angelic or spiritual being that acts as your "stop sign." Avoid the worst of the *transmediumship* gift — which involves allowing external energies into your body — by *channeling* or listening only to the wisdom, diagnostics, or healing energies acceptable to your gatekeeper or your own spirit. When you are working the pathways, answers will come in words or tones. You will excel at using commands on the power pathway or tones on any pathway to heal concerns. The power of words and tones can also summon healing energies on any of the pathways.

Chakra Six: Visual sympathy. You perceive psychic information in pictures, symbols, colors, or shapes. Called *clairvoyance* or clear seeing, this gift is perhaps the most reliable for energy mapping — and well worth cultivating no matter who you are! Images can be viewed within your head or drawn on paper to illustrate the origins of disease; vibrational qualities of the causes of the cancer; and energies, colors, tones, or elements that will heal. For best results, ask to see through your higher self or spirit.

Chakra Seven: Spiritual sympathy. This is an ideal access point for spirit contact, as you connect with your higher self, the world of spirits, and the Divine through the pineal gland. Build bridges to the various worlds of higher knowledge through prayer, asking always that the Divine screen and filter data. The seventh chakra is perfect for defining truth on any pathway. Know that you can use *prophecy* — the gift of discovering what is destined or fated — to determine if a cancer can be healed, and if so, how.

Chakra Eight: Shadow sympathy. As a shaman, you connect worlds. You journey between dimensions and the various worlds of existence, calling forth powers, energies, and information. You can read the Akashic Records — recordings of all that has ever occurred — and look for curses, bindings, and other control techniques. You can work any of the pathways to search for truth and healing, but it's likely you will excel in the imagination pathway. Enter an altered state before working.

Chakra Nine: Soul sympathy. You excel at working with higher principles and concepts and can learn how to make physical reality conform to these ideals. Work on the power pathway to command energies to adapt to the highest plan. In addition, use your gift to read the language of souls. Within the ninth chakra lies all the knowledge needed to learn about your own or another's soul identity, plans, symbols, desires, and relationships. Check whether cords, curses, and other energetic contracts compromise any of your gifts. (For details about these, see the insert and also my book, *Advanced Chakra Healing*.)

Chakra Ten: Natural sympathy. Nature is one of the most important teachers and models for healing. All of nature is alive with energies, spirits, and truths for healing. Learn to read the signs of nature as did the shamans of yore, looking to animals, planets, and plants for diagnosis. Then, on the elemental pathway, use the properties of nature for healing, whether in diet or for divining. Call upon energies such as the elemental beings or faery helpers to assist you, then reach into the power pathway to infuse your work with supernatural forces. You can learn how to accept the properties or nutrients of anything in nature directly into your body for healing and information.

Chakra Eleven: Force sympathy. The eleventh chakra connects with the eleventh auric field. Through this chakra you receive knowledge of the forces that might be keeping you ill or those that can provide healing. Through this auric field, you command movement of these and other forces to meet your goals. Practice using the elements, spirits of the elements, and spiritual energetic forces of the power pathway to work for you.

Continuing to Develop Intuition

Here are some actions, experiences, and qualities that can help you transform your psychic abilities into intuitive faculties.

Cultivation: Take classes and read books. Practice in daily life and assess your skills. Work with a psychotherapist if you feel blocked, as trauma can sometimes block our gifts.

Prayer: Praying is talking to the Divine. Communicating with the Divine expands your psychic parameters. Connection to the Divine increases safety and allows for healthy psychic boundaries, ensuring that the messages you will receive are valid.

Meditation: Meditation invites the Divine to respond to you. When meditating, you clear brain chatter and open to wisdom from higher sources. If you ask a specific question, you may not obtain a reply during your meditative practice, but be patient; you will at some point.

Contemplation: Contemplation involves basking in the presence of the Spirit, the immutable presence of the Divine. Love heals all and it is everywhere. This healing presence automatically smoothes your chakras and auric fields.

In essence:

- Prayer is like calling the Divine on the phone
- Meditation involves awaiting a response from the Divine
- Contemplation is like inviting the Divine to visit

Intensity: Pay attention to your strong inspirations or gut senses. The more powerful the message, the greater the chance that it is important. If you receive advice three or more times, either psychically or in daily life, you should probably heed the wisdom. Psychic information sent or received consciously or unconsciously by someone in a highly emotional state, during a physical trauma, or when undergoing a profound spiritual experience is more likely to attract attention. Use this knowledge in reverse, and intensely communicate your needs to others and the Divine when you are ill, or if you want to receive attention.

Religious or spiritual study: Study after study shows that people are more likely to receive spiritual revelation if they believe in God—the Divine, by any other name. Likewise, the type of psychic phenomenon you experience will fit with your cultural and religious icons. If you believe in Christ, you're more apt to be visited by him than by the Lakota healer Black Elk.

Desire: We must want something 110 percent to really get it! The second and sixth chakras are involved in this manifesting truth, as the feelings from your second chakra instruct your sixth chakra to open to an infrared energy that can manifest. Simultaneously, your seventh chakra can pull physical energy upward from your first and spin your sixth chakra desires into the universe. Mean what you say, say what you mean, and act accordingly. This combination blends the best of the physical and psychic means for healing and manifesting.

Illness: Don't be dismayed if you are learning how to access your intuition when you are ill. Use your illness. Both mental and physical illness or trauma decreases your reliance on the five senses. It's actually easier to tap higher brain waves or achieve an altered state of consciousness when ill. Go into your illness to do your energy mapping; don't wait until you feel better.

Psychological repair: Weakened psychological, social, or emotional boundaries increase your susceptibility to psychic information and can attract disturbing or inaccurate sources. If the psychic information is providing you with negative insights, work with a therapist or a spiritual counselor. Never reinforce your agitated assumptions about the world.

Closeness: The more intimate you are with someone, dead or alive, the greater your chance of communicating psychically with them or others. Consider the numerous studies of twins. Most sets of twins relate psychically. Their psychic connections correlate, whether they live near each other or not. Think of how many people you know who remain in communication with or receive visitations from deceased loved ones. Use your sense of closeness to figure out which spirits or people to trust or not and those with whom you could establish healthy psychic links.

Near death experience (NDE) or high spiritual attainment: Individuals who have been clinically dead and returned to life test as significantly more psychic than non-NDEers, as they are called. A growing body of evidence shows the same of highly spiritual individuals. The two types of individuals are revealed to be biochemically different, according to brain research. If you've had an NDE, use the gifts that were awakened at that time. Otherwise, continue climbing the sky toward spiritual awareness, for you then reach the stars!

Previous psychic experiences: Research also suggests that once you or a family member has had a psychic experience you are more likely to have another one. Sometimes certain psychic gifts seem to run in families. The idea of "the sight" is well known throughout Great Britain, for instance, as is the ability to hear or see ghosts. There is power in both belief and desire that creates psychic experiences. Remember your previous psychic experiences and identify which chakras were used. Interview family members to uncover familial strengths.

With your psychic gifts attuned, you are ready to energy map and shift heal on any of the pathways. The special insert that follows shows you how to energy map. It outlines energy information you'll need to know, then provides healing techniques usable on any of the pathways.

special insert

A Quick Reference Guide to Pathway Ideas and Techniques

There is information useful to all pathways, as well as diagnostic and healing techniques you can use for energy mapping on every pathway. This insert can serve as a reference for you as you energy map. It covers the following basics:

These first five sections provide background information for energy healing and energy mapping. This material serves as the basis for your energy work.

Following the section on Energy Absorption Issues are exercises and techniques that you can use for energy healing. You can refer back to the first five sections of this chapter for background information on the following topics:

Energy work can be daunting for those of us unfamiliar with it, or who lack practice. It's helpful to remember that you have been working energetically your entire life! You are made of energy. Your energy organs have been busily managing your bodies and welfare without your conscious awareness. Think of the gains you can make by tinkering with your energy system just a little bit.

Like any task, energy healing is easiest if you are relaxed and serene. Before beginning any energy-based exercise, take a few minutes to clear your mind and calm your body. First, clear the space around you. Literally. Get rid of any clutter surrounding the area you are going to work within, and set the lighting for your own comfort. Turn off your cell phone and check for potential intruders. Can you snatch a few minutes away from the kids, or any other demands that might interfere? Now take a few deep breaths, and concentrate on relaxing each part of your body, beginning with your feet. Feel your feet. Imagine that they are planted in the ground, anchored securely within the earth. Clench and then release each major muscle group in your body, toe to head, and then with a final big breath, ask the Divine to assign guides to attend you. As you open to negotiating reality with your intuition, remind yourself that you have been intuitive throughout your life, relying on your sense of inner knowing to manage everything from relationships to the cooking of dinner. (Don't blame your intuition if you habitually burn the latter, however.) Now you can begin to work energetically.

The first time you work with energy, you might experience any number of reactions. A lot of people feel tingling, or sensations of hot or cold. This means that you are opening, receiving, or releasing energies, in that order respectively. You might undergo various feelings, memory flashbacks, strange thoughts, dream-like awareness, or other sensations. Often there's a backlog of emotions, memories, and thoughts that floods out when we open the doors of our chakras. You might feel suddenly afraid or judgmental of the task at hand. This commonly occurs when someone becomes close to an issue or memory that is frightening, but important. Or you might feel nothing at all.

If nothing happens in the moment, observe your feelings, dreams, and thoughts over the next few days. Chances are you'll experience some changes. Chakras are physical organs, and the body often releases or attracts energy gradually. Most energy workers warn their clients about a "healing crisis" that typically occurs within ten days of an energy session. Unblocked emotions, long-standing issues, repressed beliefs, and crusty judgments, when invited forth, can sometimes create the sense of a physical or emotional catastrophe. Think of it. Let's say that you just unblocked long-standing grief, which has been stored in the lungs. Guess what you'll be doing for a few days? Crying! You might even get a cold, as most emotions attach to organisms. Release the grief and you get rid of a virus that's been living in your lungs.

Chakra Diagnosis and Healing

Most of your pathway work will be accomplished through the chakras. Within this section are basic details on the following areas:

- Vibrational Considerations
- Chakra Work with Form, Spin, and Speed
- Healing Infrastructure with Shape, Spin, and Speed
- Chakra Diagnosis by Color
- Healing with Symbology: Geometric and Number Symbols
- Tone Diagnosis and Healing

Vibrational Considerations

There are many considerations when working with the chakras vibrationally, most relating to the properties of energy that we explored in chapter 3. Two important issues involving differentiating between a chakra's front and back sides, as well as its inner and outer wheels.

Each in-body chakra begins in the center of the spine. From this center point, it generates a vortex in the front and back of the body, forming a chakra front versus a back side. In general, the front side regulates energies affecting your conscious, everyday behavior while the back side manages energies regarding your unconscious programming and spiritual beliefs. Chakras eight through twelve are not anchored in the body, but are considered to have front and back sides as these chakras spin energies that affect the front versus back side parts of your body and energy system.

It's easy to distinguish the front rather than back side of an in-body chakra. The front of a chakra spins in front of your body; the back side emanates in back of your body! Determining the front versus back side of an out-of-body chakra is just as simple. The front side generates energies that affect the front of your body and the front side of your in-body chakras, while the opposite is true for the out-of-body back sides.

Chakras also have an inner versus outer wheel. The inner wheel runs energies formulated from your subconscious or unconscious, as well as spiritual beliefs. The outer wheel generates energies formulated from conscious decisions that, in turn, affect your daily actions. The inner wheel is more likely than the outer to be affected by events originating in your soul, experienced in past lives, or passed down from ancestors, while the outer wheel reflects reactions to and beliefs about this-life experiences, such as those involving your family of origin, culture, or personal actions.

There are several ways to find the front versus back sides of your chakras, as well as the inner and outer wheels. Psychically, you can apply your intuition to see the chakras in your mind's eye, sense the operation of your chakras and their separate parts, or listen for tones. A chakra's front side and outer wheel will be a little higher pitched than their back side and inner wheel counterparts, as the former generates energies that are less dense. Physically, you can work with a pendulum as described in the section "Chakra Work with Form, Spin, and Speed," later in this chapter. Know that it's much more difficult to use a pendulum to find the inner and outer wheel; therefore, it's easiest to work psychically. Typically, you are measuring the outer wheel when working with a pendulum.

Following is a brief reference to help you work with the different structures of a chakra.

Front and back side: Your twelve major chakras each have a front and a back side. In general, the front side processes your conscious and daily needs; the back side processes your unconscious and primal programs.

Left and right: The left sides of your body and your chakras process information stereotypically considered feminine — feelings, the unconscious, issues about receiving, and spirituality. The right sides of your body and chakras deal with stereotypically masculine energies — those concerning your everyday life and accomplishments, and issues about giving, conquering, and action.

Infrastructure: Chakras each have an inner and an outer wheel. Both should be spinning in rhythm with each other. The inner wheel regulates the unconscious energies controlled by that chakra and can connect you to various planes and zones of existence, other worlds, and other dimensions. The outer wheel is your energetic contact between these other realities and the external world. It is primarily affected by your here-and-now, conscious life and thoughts.

Shape: There are two aspects to shape: *spin* and *form*.

- *Spin:* Chakras ideally maintain even spins in both the internal and external wheels. Both wheels usually move clockwise, pulling necessary energy from various planes and worlds to enable a healthy life. Reverse or counterclockwise spins sometimes indicate a release of toxins. A continual reverse spin anywhere but in the inner wheel of the eighth chakra, or in some of the spaces of the eighth auric field, indicates disease and a loss of necessary life energy.

- *Form* references the various geometric and other forms in which energy can appear, as well the types of forms that can affect energy. Cancer cells, for instance, have abnormal forms in comparison with healthy cells. The chakras affecting and affected by cancer will also possess abnormal forms. The normal form for a chakra is circular.

A circular, evenly spinning chakra is healthy and functioning normally. Imbalances usually indicate problems that are negatively or positively charged. You can diagnose the problems underlying various cancers by observing a chakra's shape and sometimes hold a healing using other shapes.

Speed: In general, the lower the chakra, the more slowly it should be moving. When wheels within a certain chakra are moving at contrary speeds, out of rhythm with each other, or out of rhythm with the other chakras, you must evaluate for bad programming or disease.

Color: Psychically, each chakra appears in a certain color. Color is one measure of vibration and also of information. We'll be looking at the typical colors associated with each chakra. You will need to know these in order to evaluate the presence or type of cancer and to use color to heal this cancer.

Symbology: Encoded in each chakra are symbols and numbers holding that chakra in alignment with its core spiritual programming. Unfortunately, the energetics of these symbols can be warped through life's negative influences. You can determine the injury to a chakra, a strand of DNA, an oncogene, or any other integral element of cancer by evaluating symbols and numbers; in turn, you can amend problems using symbology.

Tones: An auditory person has only to listen to a chakra to evaluate it for health. Likewise, he or she can command change through words, music, tones, or sounds. Tones are vibratory. A cancer will make the chakra that governs that area sound "off tone." *In energy mapping, the reader is listening to the chakras, not the actual cancer.* If you can retune the chakra to the body, you can alter the negative programming of the cancer cell.

To determine the form, spin, or speed of a chakra using this instrument, the subject (or yourself, using someone else as a tester) can either lie down or sit in a chair. It's easiest to evaluate front and back side chakra spins when someone is lying down.

Hold the pendulum about anywhere from several inches to a foot over a chakra center. You will feel a subtle tug of energy when connecting with the vortex. Keep your hand steady. If linked with the chakra, the pendulum will slowly begin to swing. Within a few moments, this swing will take form and pick up speed. When the movement is stabilized, you can evaluate it for function or dysfunction.

A healthy chakra will cause the pendulum to spin in a broad, full circle at a measured speed. What's the best way to determine if a chakra looks this way? Play around until you find a chakra that is off. The swing might arc to the left or the right, make a straight line horizontally or vertically, spin in hypo- or hyperdrive, swoop in a tight or gigantic loop, or maybe just remain at a standstill. These off-swings are meaningful, and can indicate the presence or nature of disease. Having seen a dysfunctional chakra, you can now also figure out which chakras are healthier.

Techniques for psychically evaluating swing are similar to those provided in the section "Vibrational Considerations," earlier in this insert, in reference to discerning the front and back sides and inner and outer wheels of the chakras. In general, a visual sensitive will peer into a chakra for pictures that illustrate a spin. A kinesthetic will sense or feel disturbances. And the verbally gifted will listen for tones that seem distorted or aberrant. If you are verbal, it's best to first assess the general harmonic of your body. To determine your personal harmonic, you can use the exercise "Keying into Your Personal Harmonic" mentioned in chapter 7 in this book and described in-depth in *Advanced Chakra Healing.* This harmonic can serve as your baseline for evaluating chakra health. Tones that are too high pitched in comparison to the baseline, for instance, can indicate a chakra spin that is too fast. Tones that are too low might reveal a spin that is too slow.

Chakra Work with Form, Spin, and Speed

You can evaluate a chakra for its various functions and for broad movement using a pendulum or your psychic senses. A pendulum is any small object on a chain or a string. Hold it a few inches over a chakra to check out the configurations of the chakra.

Evaluating Form Here are some basic meanings of the general chakra shapes as perceived with the pendulum or through psychic vision.

- *Round:* Healthy and balanced.
- *Lacking substance on right* (from subject's perspective): Oriented toward unconscious programming, emotions, right-brain creative, but lacking action and follow-through.
- *Lacking substance on left:* Geared toward consciousness behavior and actions, left-brain analytic, but lacking creativity and intuition.
- *Lacking substance on bottom:* More spiritual than practical.
- *Lacking substance on top:* More practical than spiritual.

Correct the situation by shifting energies until the chakra is balanced. Use a symbol to hold this new shape; a cross of equal lines always works. I also recommend surrounding this cross with a circle. In this form, it actually mirrors the Celtic cross of the British Isles, an ancient and mystical symbol for protection.

Evaluating Spin A chakra should hold a solid, even spin. From the point of view of the pendulum holder, a healthy chakra front side spin will cause the pendulum to move clockwise and to the right. A healthy chakra back side swing will actually appear counterclockwise! To make measurement easier, I am describing how to evaluate chakra health from the front sides only. You will have to reverse the description to analyze the back sides. The front side and back sides should be moving in the same direction. Clockwise spins usually indicate health, unless they are moving too quickly. A counterclockwise spin often shows a blockage or a misperception, unless that chakra is temporarily detoxifying. However, the eighth chakra's inner wheel should be moving counterclockwise frequently, as it functions as a central clearinghouse. In general, you want all chakras opened the same amount and spinning at about the same rate. This indicates a balanced system.

Following are the meanings of spins in both the inner and outer wheels.

- *Round, uniform, and even swing, clockwise:* Healthy and functioning.
- *Round, uniform, and even swing, counterclockwise:* Attempting to create health or balance by processing or clearing negative energy.
- *Nonuniform or uneven swing, counterclockwise:* Chakra is blocked and unable to clear itself.
- *Elliptical or straight line in a vertical direction:* Developed but impractical spiritual views, closed to real-life perspective, or unwilling to take action.
- *Elliptical or straight line in a horizontal direction:* Practical but lacking spiritual perspective, closed to big picture or divine assistance.
- *Elliptical or straight line, swinging to the right (of the subject):* Oriented toward action and the day to day, known as the masculine perspective, but lacking the emotional or spiritual, known as the feminine perspective.
- *Elliptical or straight line, swinging to the left (of the subject):* Oriented toward inspirational, feminine, or intuitive influences but lacking practical, grounding action.

- *Not moving or nearly still:* Indicates a closed chakra. Function is shut down. This is a good place to look for the block or cause of a presenting issue.
- *Large swing:* Usually means very open, healthy, and functioning. If too large and imbalanced in comparison to other chakras, it means the chakra is overstrained and overfunctioning. Figure out which chakra this one is compensating for.
- *Small swing:* Underfunctioning; must be cleared and opened.

Evaluating Speed The lower the chakra, the slower both wheels should be moving. The inner wheel usually moves exactly twice the speed of the outer wheel and, except for the eighth chakra, in the same direction. Here are other diagnostic tips.

- *Wheel too slow:* Indicates damage from previous overuse, exhaustion, fatigue, blocks, strongholds, and probably repressed memories or feelings. Often reflects depressed or electron-charged energies.
- *Wheel too fast:* Indicates current overuse; overstrain; acting to compensate for a weaker chakra or chakra wheel; or a desire to escape certain life events, people, feelings, or issues. Could be an attempt to release negative energy. Often reflects anxious or proton-charged energies.
- *Outer wheel fast, inner wheel slow:* Lack of spiritual, emotional, intuitive, or creative drive or perspective; underdeveloped beliefs, feelings, or spiritual sense; overconcern with physical appearance.
- *Outer wheel slow, inner wheel fast:* Lacking action, commitment to follow through, physical drive, or energy; overconcern with spiritual or psychic matters; fear of moving into the world; exhaustion in the physical.
- *Wheels out of synch:* Inner beliefs and needs don't match with outer reality or action.

Healing Infrastructure with Shape, Spin, and Speed

Consult a medical professional to determine the exact cause of all problems. Only then should you consider using vibration to change speed, spin, or form for healing. Here's a list of five basic methods for vibration healing, followed by details you can draw on in using the first three.

- Infuse with color. Taking out discoloration and incorporating the correct color can change speed, spin, or shape.
- Use symbology. In the center of each chakra is a symbol representing the elemental program of the chakra. Remove negative symbols, repair injured yet accurate symbols, or insert supportive symbols.
- Use toning. Tones can spin out a problem or help infuse a solution.
- Examine power levels on the elemental pathway.
- Assess beliefs, feelings, and strongholds.

Chakra Diagnosis by Color

You can diagnose based on the colors you would expect in each chakra when healthy, as shown in the following table.

Chakra	**Color**	**Meaning of Color**
One	Red	Passion
Two	Orange	Feelings and creativity
Three	Yellow	Wisdom and power
Four	Green	Healing
Five	Blue	Communication and guidance
Six	Purple	Vision
Seven	White	Spirituality
Eight	Black	Karma: the effect of the past
Nine	Gold	Soul purpose and unity with others
Ten	Earth tones	Relationship to the environment
Eleven	Pink	Transmutation (of negative to positive and vice versa)
Twelve	Clear	Link of human with Divine

Harmful Coloration When colors inside the chakra or body are off, you can use this information to identify what is causing the problem. Here are the meanings of various altered colors.

Added red tones	Overstimulates passion, anger, ego, or survival fears.
Added orange tones	Creates emotionalism or hyperactivity.
Added yellow tones	Overemphasizes certain mental ideas or beliefs to create falsehoods or judgments.
Added green tones	Overstimulates drive for relationships, codependency, and perceived need to heal what doesn't need healing.
Added pink tones	Can create a sense of love where it doesn't exist.
Added blue tones	Causes perceived need to obtain more and more guidance or to overexplain oneself.
Added purple tones	Causes compulsive planning or difficulties in seeing or sorting out choices.
Added white tones	Overstimulates sense of spirituality and deemphasizes the need for power and action.
Added black tones	Imbalances spiritual energies with an emphasis on power. Can cause powerlessness, emotionalism, or greed.
Added gold tones	Causes excessive idealism and a resulting loss of hope.
Added silver tones	Creates susceptibility to psychic sources.
Added brown tones	Muddies the waters and results in confusion, hyperpracticality, and mundane obsessions.
Added gray tones	Shadows or covers an issue, causing lack of clarity.
Neutralizing	Erasing intensity creates emptiness and powerlessness. Voodoo and mind control use these methods.

Imposing	Forcing a color over someone else's, thus achieving control over the other person. This is also called creating an "overlay."
Blotching	Creates inconsistency, making it hard for a victim to rely on him- or herself.

Missing Colors and the Missing Self If you perceive empty spaces where there ought to be color, shape, or form, some aspect of the self is probably fragmented and held either in another aspect of the self or elsewhere. *Possession* occurs when an aspect of something else or some external energy lies within your own field. *Recession* involves subjugation of an aspect of self in another entity. An exercise for dealing with these issues appears in this insert.

Coloring Your Healing Each color listed represents a different type of energy. Adding these colors to a chakra produces the intended effect.You can add colors psychically by picturing the desired hue and infusing it into the depleted area, sensing the needed color in the weak area, or imagining a tone that invokes the required color and humming it in your mind. As well, you can add the missing color to your wardrobe, household, or office.

- Red — Life energy
- Orange — Creativity and feelings
- Yellow — Intellect
- Green — Healing
- Pink/rose — Love
- Blue — Communication
- Purple — Vision, clarification of choices, and decision results
- White — Divine will, spiritual destiny
- Black — Power for movement, force behind change
- Gold — Harmony
- Silver — Transference of energy from one place to another
- Brown — Practicality and grounding

Healing with Symbology: Geometric and Number Symbols

To conduct symbol diagnosis and healing, examine the center of the chakra to see what symbol is determining the current state of disrepair. An off symbol will look twisted, skewed, or misshapen in some way that alters it from wholeness (hence I use the term "altered" to describe these symbols in the following chart). Then return to the spirit-enhancing lists to identify which symbol to replace it with.

Geometric Symbols

Harmful

· Altered Circle	Breaks positive relationships or creates harmful ones.
· Altered Square	Is used to overthrow or topple systems.
· Altered Rectangle	Imprisons or exposes to danger.
· Altered Triangle	Creates illness, disease, imbalance, and death.
· Altered Spiral	Forces abrupt endings, cessation of cycles or rhythms.
· Altered Five-Pointed Star	Stifles, contains, suffocates, makes base.
· Altered Six-Pointed Star	Causes stuckness, despair, and depression.
· Altered Cross	Accentuates ego or causes extreme dejection.
· An "X"	Is evil or anticonsciousness.

Spirit-Enhancing

· Circle	Wholeness
· Square	Foundation
· Rectangle	Protection
· Triangle	Preservation and immortality

• Spiral	Creation and cycles
• Five-Pointed Star	Alchemy and movement
• Six-Pointed Star	Resurrection
• Cross	Human-Divine connection and spiritual protection

Number Symbols Numerical symbols can actually be psychically perceived as numbers that appear in the chakras. Sometimes a kinesthetic person will sense and "just know" a number, while a verbal sensitive will hear a sequence of tones that can be added to a number. While spirit-enhancing numbers appear, look, or sound complete, altered numbers will appear broken or distorted, feel "off," or sound cut off or out of beat. All numbers can be perceived in a chakric center.

Harmful

• Altered One	Prevents you from reaching a conclusion.
• Altered Two	Forces unhealthy liaisons; keeps victims stuck on powerless side of the power levels.
• Altered Three	Causes chaos.
• Altered Four	Imprisons or creates craziness.
• Altered Five	Creates trickery or delusion.
• Altered Six	Causes confusion and disorder, convincing the victim to choose evil. The number of the lie.
• Altered Seven	Establishes doubt about the Creator's very existence.
• Altered Eight	Stifles learning and forces the recycling of harmful patterns.
• Altered Nine	Instills terror and fear about change; keeps victims stuck in the eight.
• Altered Ten	Prevents new beginnings and seeks to make victims continue the old ways.

- Altered Eleven — Obliterates self-esteem and seeks to keep victims from accepting their humanity.
- Altered Twelve — Disavows forgiveness and casts shadows over human goodness.

Spirit-Enhancing

One	Beginnings. Represents the highest form, the Creator.
Two	Pairing and duality. Reflects that everything in the material universe is made of opposites, which are the same. A two splits unity but also holds two ones in unity.
Three	The number of creation, which lies between and emanates from a beginning and an ending.
Four	Foundation and stability. The number of complete balance — consider the four-legged stool.
Five	Direction setting. Space for making decisions. Represents the human figure, able to go in every direction at once or to travel at will.
Six	Choices. The presence of light and dark, good and evil, and gifts of love, as offered through free will.
Seven	Spiritual principles. The Divine. The number of love and action that produces grace. Key number of the third dimension.
Eight	Infinity. Recurring patterns and karma. Path of recycling. The number of knowledge.
Nine	Change. Elimination of what was. Ending of the cycles of the eight. The highest single-digit number, nine can erase error and evil and bring us to a new beginning.
Ten	New life. Release of the old and acceptance of the new. This number of physical matter can record the heavenly on earth.
Eleven	Acceptance of what has been and what will be. Release of personal mythology. Opening to divine powers.
Twelve	Mastery over human drama. Becoming okay with being fully human and seeing the power in it. Mystery of the human as divine.

Geometric and Number Combinations Certain geometric symbols derive extra power from their connection with a particular number. For example:

Number	**Geometric Symbol(s)**
One	Dot or circle
Two	Horizontal line
Three	Triangle
Four	Cross with arms of equal length; also an equilateral quadrangle
Five	Pentagon; also a pentagram
Six	Equilateral hexagram
Seven	Equilateral septangle; also a rainbow
Eight	Equilateral octagon
Nine	Three equilateral triangles
Ten	Circle with a cross of eight arms; also a square with a circle in the middle
Eleven	Parallel lines
Twelve	A corona or rising sun with twelve lines; also the lotus

Tone Diagnosis and Healing

All musical notes hold a vibration and create different results. The human body is attuned to the A note, as explained in *Advanced Chakra Healing: Energy Medicine*. This means that all of the body's physical and energetic systems will balance with A from the core of a chakra outward, especially if our heritage is Western. Eastern cultures adapt from a variety of other chords, tending toward more flat (or sharp), atonal, or chromatic as base line. Various scientific research, however, is proposing that the entire universe began and will end on an A, so I believe that all life is sensitive to this basic note.

Tones can heal and also can harm. Off-tones throw your body out of kilter. Correct tones blend with your core harmonic and keep you strong. Listen for tones for diagnosis and also to check which ones will enable a healing.

Here are the meanings of the basic tonal vibrations.

Whole Notes

A	Of spirit	Attunes human to divine nature, your human self to your spiritual self
B	Of mind	Attunes your Lower and Middle Mind to the Higher Mind
C	Of feelings	Attunes your human feelings to spiritual feelings
D	Of body	Attunes your physical body, condition, or material needs to your spiritual body, gifts, or manifesting abilities
E	Of love	Attunes whatever is out of love to unconditional divine love
F	Of miracles	Attunes any aspect of your being to the spiritual forces needed at that time, breaking through duality into the miraculous
G	Of grace	Delivers grace, which is divine love and divine power, to the situation at hand

Sharps and Flats Sharps bring the spiritual into material reality. An F sharp, for instance, activates that part of your internal spirit that links you with the force you now require. Flats allow release. A G flat, for instance, which is the same as an F sharp, pushes out any negative or evil forces preventing your spiritual destiny. The difference between working with a sharp and a flat is intention. If you desire to get rid of something, think flat; to attract something, think sharp.

Core Tones Many esoteric groups work with a C-based system of musical scales. I point out that there are two versions of the scales. The first is octave-based, in which notes are repeated in eights. The second counts in fifths; this is the model that I believe underlies the Primary Grid, alchemy, and the divine pathway. I start fifths with an A, then merge the idea of the octaves into it for elemental-based healing.

Basic Chakra

Tones	*My Theory*	*Esoteric Theory*
First chakra	A	C
Second chakra	B	D
Third chakra	C	E
Fourth chakra	D	F
Fifth chakra	E	G
Sixth chakra	F	A
Seventh chakra	G	B
Eighth chakra	A	C
Ninth chakra	B	D
Tenth chakra	C	E
Eleventh chakra	D	F

A more personalized way to figure out tonal healing is to establish your own baseline. Please see chapter 8, on the power pathway, and conduct the exercise "Keying into Your Personal Harmonic."

Other Energy Bodies Vital to Pathway Healing

There are dozens of energy bodies. Each pathway has energy bodies unique to itself; a few of these are briefly described in the chapters about each pathway. The remainder you can study in *Advanced Chakra Healing*. The auric field, energy egg, and etheric mirror, however, interconnect all the pathways and are important to know about.

Your Auric Field

While your chakras run the "you inside of you," your auric field regulates the "you outside of you." There are twelve basic bands in your auric field, just as there are twelve chakras. These two sets of organs are paired. The first chakra, for instance, is partnered with the first band of the auric field, and so on. Because of this partnership, changes you make through your chakras are automatically translated into your auric field, and vice versa.

The auric field is important for setting boundaries that protect you and screen information. Information has to pass through the parameters of your field to make it into your chakras and therefore your body. Communiqués sent from your chakras must pass through the screen of your aura to be delivered into the world. Regarding cancer, it's very important to establish the correct relationship between these two energy bodies. You might really want to heal from cancer but be carrying a program in your auric field that refuses to communicate your intense desire to the world. This will make it hard to attract the kinds of doctors and supporters needed to gain optimum assistance. Perhaps you're undergoing chemotherapy and it actually wipes out the cancer. Unless your auric field "breathes" and passes out toxins, however, the poisonous aftereffects of the chemotherapy will remain in your body and can potentially create yet a new and different cancer.

Your Energy Egg

The *energy egg* is an electromagnetic body that penetrates and surrounds your twelve chakras and auric bands. It creates the outer rim of your human energy system, psychically appearing as a pulsating, three-layer field of incandescent energies. Working with the energy egg for healing helps achieve several goals. Through the energy egg, you can:

- Clear the programs or beliefs held in the subconscious and unconscious that might be causing illness and problems

- Connect your higher conscious to your everyday conscious, so you can attract your highest desires
- Diagnose and then release the negative information and energies causing your illness
- Attract the spiritual energies or "waves" that create real and permanent changes in health and happiness

To work with your energy egg, you must understand the structure of this energy body and how it works with your chakras and auric fields in relationship with your programming.

The Structure of Your Energy Egg There are three layers to an energy egg. You can connect to any of these layers at will through your pineal gland, but you will most likely link only with the innermost layer unless you have achieved a relatively high state of consciousness. This *first layer of the energy egg* relays information-energy between your body and inner psyche and the world at large. This first layer is responsible for alerting the world about the messages of your subconscious and for attracting the needs programmed into your brain. Deep psychological, emotional, or otherwise challenging issues are observable in this layer; these will limit your ability to allow energies from the other two layers into your physical self. This layer can be contacted through the pineal gland, but also through the twelfth auric field and chakra, the latter of which connects into thirty-two secondary points of energy in your body.

The *second layer of the energy egg* looks psychically like a thin line of energy that intersperses black energies and white energies. This layer attracts that which you imagine within your unconscious. You could call it the layer of wish making and dreaming. If your programming is warped, you will access energies that deter you from destiny, or form fantasies that are unrealistic. If your use of the second layer is healthy, your twelfth chakra and auric field enable the manifestation of desires into your everyday life.

The *third layer of the energy egg* is an incandescent, shimmering body of energy that interconnects the outer rim of the twelfth chakra and auric field and the spiritual realms that lie beyond the human self. This layer attracts only that which fits your highest spiritual needs and purposes; it is therefore connected to what you could call your highest consciousness. It can actually call energies into your life that don't yet exist on this planet, but which will benefit you and other people. The possibility for producing physical and emotional miracles lies in working this layer.

Your Etheric Mirror

The *etheric mirror* copies your etheric body, which comprises the tenth auric field and first auric field. The etheric body doubles your physical body; both can be damaged by life experiences, and over time these two energy bodies become different from each other. The etheric mirror, on the other hand, holds the correct and perfect codes for your physical and energetic body. Through it you access accurate DNA patterns and use intention, vibrational methods, or various techniques according to pathway, to translate these energies directly into the body.

I also call this the Christ body, as it has seemingly magical healing powers. Using the term "Christ" refers to the ancient mystical principle of the human and the divine being interconnected. We each have a Christ nature and the potential for being fully human and divine simultaneously.

Your Energy Fields

Several energy fields are critical to the healing process.

Etheric fields surround every quantum, cell, organ, and living being, as well as many inanimate energies. Etheric materials usually vibrate at octave levels above their corresponding physical cousins. They can generate information that is slower or faster than the speed of light, and they often "catch" information that can cause diseases such as cancer before the physical body incorporates this information.

Programs for cancer are often first received and held in the etheric field. Acute or constant stress can force the etheric field to dump the cancer vibration into the body, hence the appearance of "overnight" or sudden cancers. The etheric field around a single cell or cellular nucleus can also be vulnerable to sudden stress. When the etheric wall crumbles, the genes can become damaged, lose their rhythm, and therefore mutate. You can often read the material of the etheric mirror to determine whether an etheric field, energy body, or part of your physical body is uniform with its ideal.

The most basic field is your body's *electromagnetic field.* The heart, brain, and central nervous system are the three most vital perpetuators of your internal electrical system. The heart generates thousands of times more electrical energy than does your brain (the master of the central nervous system, which includes your spine). These three organs or systems interact, sending and receiving information from the external environment into your internal environment, and vice versa. As well, every single cell pulses with electrical information, which serves as a conduit for passing information. Through your electrical system, all cells are able to "reach through" the physical walls of the body and receive direct messages from the world outside of the body. The tiniest atom within a cell nucleus can speak to the stars, because information can vibrate everywhere, all at once.

Electricity run through a conduit generates a magnetic field—hence the term *electromagnetic field.* Every part of your body vibrates electrically, and therefore produces a magnetic field. The auric field is really a vibrating set of magnetic fields (which hold some electrical properties) both around and, to an extent, within your physical body. This means that the energies that affect and are generated by your auric field will vibrate throughout every part of your body.

A lack of vitality in your magnetic field will greatly weaken the affected auric band, but also your entire auric field, making you more susceptible to disease. Too much electrical energy in your auric field, in comparison with your magnetic field, and you'll attract negative energies — such as others' emotions or issues — into your body.

Morphogenetic fields convey information from one person or one group to another. There are morphogenetic fields connecting all animals, the various species, all humans, and people within a country or members of a family. Cancers, or the vibrations causing them, can be shared through various morphogenetic fields; this accounts in part for some of the cancers that are specific to ethnic or family types.

The *Vivaxis* is a word coined by naturopath Judy Jacka to describe the various networks of fields that run through and around the planetary globe. Some of these energetic fields connect the earth to other planets and planes; others link us to the electromagnetic fields on this planet. Many cancers are caused or impacted by geopathic stress (a concept introduced in chapter 2). Fields generated from microwaves, radio stations, power lines, nuclear power plants, and more cause vibrational damage to our generic fields and create the conditions for malignancy.

The fields listed here, plus others, are part of what I call the *Secondary Grid*, an interlocking network of energetic lines, fields, and forces that cause duality on this planet and in our bodies. Duality is the belief that there are oppositional energies. If someone perceives herself to be a victim all the time, for instance, she will be unlikely to contact the energies that can make her more powerful. In reference to cancer, if you believe yourself to be a victim of cancer, it will be difficult for you to also see yourself as a victor of the cancer. In contrast, we can also choose to operate on the *Primary Grid*, a star-studded formation of spiritual truths that occupy the divine pathway.

Part of the Secondary Grid is a series of power levels and power fields that relate to the inception of strongholds in your body. *Power levels* are consciousness waves that hold two dualistic notions together. They can captivate your thoughts and energies and keep you imprisoned in your mental and emotional strongholds. *Power fields* are a progressive order of energetic fields that stair-step you through the human development process into owning your divinity. A complete outline of power levels and power fields is available in *Advanced Chakra Healing*.

Kundalini: The Magic Energy

Kundalini is an ancient Hindu term for the spiritualizing of the energy system and a process for unfolding your life-force energy; it is extremely important in the recovery from cancer. All cancer cells drain your basic life energy — the red-colored unit of energy that vibrates with living consciousness.

Basic life energy is a gift from the Divine; it connects your divine self with your human self. When you are drained, depleted, or discouraged, all systems in your body fail to thrive, and you may either develop a malicious disease like cancer or be too tired to combat such a disease.

The kundalini process unfolds in every pathway except the imagination pathway; when complete, it unifies the Four Pathways. In its primary stage, kundalini starts on the elemental pathway, in the first chakra for men and the second for women; it then rises through the remainder of the energy system and comes full circle. Kundalini energy empowers your entire body in line with your spirit and can therefore bring your correct harmonic into each and every part of your body — including those with cancer.

You can induce your kundalini on three of the pathways:

- On the elemental pathway, work with *serpent* or *red kundalini* to clear the body of blockage. Red kundalini is the most primary of kundalini energies; it keeps the body health and balanced.

- On the power pathway, use *golden kundalini* from above to spiritualize the red kundalini and access spiritual powers. Golden kundalini is a spiritual energy that enters from above the head. When it merges with the red kundalini, it helps your body achieve the state of health that matches your spiritual nature.
- On the divine pathway, *radiant kundalini* emanates from each and every cell, organ, and aspect of the self upon claiming Divine love. Radiant kundalini is unique to itself, though when it generates from inside of you, it joins the red and golden kundalini and therefore completely brings all aspects of your life to your highest physical and spiritual potentials.
- On the imagination pathway there is no energy, so you can't use kundalini on it. However, actions on the imagination pathway affect kundalini positively or negatively.

Entities and Energies: Invisible Help and Harm

There are invisible entities and energies that can help or harm you. The two points to understand are sourcing and interference.

Sourcing

A *source* is an origin of information or energy. *Sourcing* involves tracing a problem or issue back to the original sources, which might be people, experiences, ideas, entities, consciousnesses, or energies that have wrongly informed you.

Cancer can start with inanimate or animate sources. *Inanimate sources* aren't alive, but most generate fields and share information. A poisonous chemical is an inanimate source of cancer. It can vibrationally disrupt an already weakened cell, or even a healthy one, and disturb that cell's natural vibration enough to create mutations. *Animate sources* are beings with consciousness. They don't have to be alive. A ghost or an angel, for instance, is an animate source. Animate sources do, of course, include people. *Helpful sources* encourage the internalizing of your personal spirit in your body, whereas *harmful sources* discourage this internalization.

When working with cancer, we almost always have to source for cause. This might involve regression, hypnotherapy, dream work, or simply memory recall to find out if (and if so, where) we have taken on disruptive energies from an external source.

Sources can be positive and life enhancing, as well as harmful or destructive. All aspects of yourself are available to help with healing and manifesting, and there are countless divine-oriented sources to assist you in your healing endeavors. In the individual chapters on the pathways, I have listed the sources that are likely to be most helpful on each pathway. Among the sources listed are natural forces, natural spirits, nature spirits, the elemental beings, beings of the stars, beings of earth, natural objects, angels, masters, avatars, ascended masters, saints, spirit guides, extraterrestrials, allies, forms and powers, and ancestors.

Interference

Interference occurs when an internal or external source of energy interrupts your natural harmonic in a harmful way. Some sources will disturb your natural harmonic to benefit you: for example, to open up a new life choice or to make you aware of potential danger. I use the term *interference* to describe interruptive negative sources, such as those that cause tragedy, trauma, and disease.

There are many types of interference, and all can be involved in establishing conditions that allow cancer. The major types are entity- or consciousness-based, aspects of the self, or energetic contracts.

Interference can directly cause the conditions for cancer or attach someone to energies that can create cancer. Aneuploid materials, for instance, can be ceded at birth from interfering energies. Though contained for decades, the aneuploid material might suddenly burst into cancer when enough physical or emotional damage has been incurred from life. This same aneuploid material can be energetically programmed into the body through physical or energetic genetics. *Energy genetics* is the sharing of information that codes your energy system first and your physical system and genetics second.

Following are lists of the various types of energies that might cause, support, or enhance cancer. More detailed descriptions are provided in *Advanced Chakra Healing*.

Entity-Based or Consciousness-Based Interference

An *entity* is a being with its own unique spirit and a soul. Through its soul, an entity traverses time and space to gather experiences. Entities most likely to affect cancers include ancestors, harmful souls, hauntings (which I'll describe shortly), and living people who project an aspect of self into or around you.

Sorcery is interference from an energy, entity, or consciousness that seeks to control its subject through manipulation.

Consciousness-based interference can be group energy, such as group consciousness, or powerful ideas that brainwash people into thinking or acting a certain way. The fear of cancer in our society is actually supported by a consciousness fear.

With cancerous conditions, I also usually check for group consciousness. A *group consciousness* is a collection of thoughts that seek to influence the thoughts of others.

Aspects of the Self

A cancer source might lie no farther than the mirror. There are many, many aspects of the self to consider when looking to source cancer, but the basic ones are:

- Your spirit, which is the immutable and eternal aspect of the self
- Your soul, which carries you through time and through experience, gaining learning and wounds on the way
- Your mind, which regulates your thinking and beliefs
- Your heart, which connects all aspects of yourself through love
- Your body, which experiences all that life has to offer in order to achieve your spiritual purpose

Other aspects include the personality; the ego; inner children and innocent child; the God self, primal self, and master self; and the High, Middle, and Low Heart, Mind, and Self. Any of these could inadvertently be creating disease, blocked in such a way as to allow it, or wishing disease upon your entire person. For instance, an angry inner child, an aspect of self that is stuck in a spacetime that caused it trauma, can be generating enough negative vibrations to cause disrepair within a cell's nucleus.

The soul is frequently responsible for certain diseases, as it carries issues from lifetime to lifetime. There are several parts to the soul, including soul fragments — individual and often independently operating parts of the soul. A soul might fragment due to trauma and be therefore susceptible to (1) disease; (2) possession, the act of being taken over by another entity or energy; or (3) recession, which involves being stuck in an aspect of something or someone else. Possession and recession can occur with or through any aspect of the self. A possessing being can will cancer upon you; missing a recessed aspect of self makes you vulnerable to DNA mutations and other weaknesses.

Energetic Contracts

Energy contracts, also called *energy cords*, are agreements made between at least two entities or energies that create a negative energy exchange. Here are some of the many types of energy contracts that might underlie cancer.

A *binding* is an energy force that puts one person or entity in charge of another.

A *curse* is a binding holding a group of people in bondage. For instance, a family can be cursed with conditions that create cancer or cause the genes to turn off the tumor-suppression proteins.

A *miasm* is the product of a familial curse and an attempt to keep everyone similar within a family system. It fixes disease patterns in the etheric energy and so operates like an energetic genetic pattern, predisposing all members of a family — or certain types of family members.

A *haunting* is a ghost or entity that forces the living into certain behaviors. A haunting can't cause cancer, but it can nag you into negative behaviors — such as smoking — that can lead to cancer.

A *spell* is a binding held over an individual for control purposes. A spell can distort all or part of your harmonic and cause discord within various cells, which might then mutate into cancer.

An *energy cord* is an energy contract that keeps you connected to another person or group. You can actually pass the programming or patterning for cancer from one person to another through an energy cord. A *life energy cord* is the most dangerous, as the person on the other end assumes your life energy, which greatly lowers your body's immunity. Without life energy, your body can't maintain its harmonic and the cells gradually lose their personal frequencies. An *enigma* is a cord that ends in an attachment in your physical body, and allows someone else to either drain your life-giving energy or dump their negative energy into you. Enigmas differ from other types of cords and contracts in that there isn't a two-way flow of energy involved. Someone can simply drain your energy (or you can drain his or her energy) with no reciprocating value. *Energy markers*, which are similar to enigmas, form counterclockwise spins, usually in symbol form, that drain your vital energy from you. The difference between an energy marker and an enigma is that with an energy marker the loss of energy may or may not involve another person. You might be leaking energy, but this energy isn't necessarily going into something or someone else. It will instruct others to treat you in disrespectful or negative ways, which can result in poor care if you do have cancer.

Childhood cancers are often the product of *holds*, energetic clamps that keep the child from developing into his or her own personal self. These holds might stem from the parents or ancestry, yet are as likely to be sourced from a religion, culture, group mind, or the child him- or herself.

A *codependent contract* is one that you make with someone else that ends up doubling back on you. Codependency involves giving to someone else in order to receive what you want from him or her. The end result is inflammation in the areas absorbing another's energies and a lowered immune system from the giving away of your own energy. These are two key factors in the development and progression of cancer.

Energetically, the codependent cord forms a figure 8, with the center point located over the original cord site. You exchange energy within your own system, at a cost to all parts of your energy system wrapped into the 8. Imagine the stress on the area centering the 8! Besides the resulting weakness in this part of the body, the exchange of energies ensures the presence of unnatural and disharmonic energies in at least two areas of the body. Essentially, this is one of the ways that cancer is spread throughout the body. You will often find a primary and secondary chakra site connected by a codependent contract. As well, this transfer of energy can account for confused pH balance in the body. An area that is too acidic might receive a dump of alkaline-producing energies, and vice versa. If this occurs in an area like the chest, you might find an electron-based cancer in one breast and a proton-based cancer in the other breast. (For more information on the psychological causes of codependent contracts, please read Cathryn Taylor's books, including *The Inner Child Workbook.*)

Others' energies can give you cancer, as is often the case with cancers in the body's storage or draining areas. The breast is often a receptacle for others' relational feelings, which women might assume, thinking that they are helping the source. The lymph system acts like a garbage collection truck for both physical and psychic energies that don't match your harmonic. If constantly overloaded with misfit energies from others, your lymph system will clog and be unable to clear malignancies.

Interference can only be released once you figure out your *payoff*—the reason that some aspect of the self allowed the interference.

To learn how to look for and deal with energy contracts, refer to the descriptions of energy contracts and cords in *Advanced Chakra Healing*.

Energy Absorption Issues

As I've stressed, energies that you pick up from others can cause cancer or create the conditions for it. Others' energies don't coordinate within your own system. Intense energies or those absorbed over time can eventually distort your DNA or disturb the cellular reproduction. Internalized energies can also keep your body from responding to an immune-system crisis, blocking help from getting where it needs to go. Here are the different types of energies that you can absorb and tips on how to recognize this problem.

Feelings

There are five main feeling groups or constellations: anger, sadness, happiness, fear, and disgust. You must deal with your own feelings to heal from cancer, but you won't get anywhere trying to heal someone else's emotions! There are many ways to know if you have taken on others' feelings (these are described in *Advanced Chakra Healing*). The easiest determinant is to ask your intuitive self to separate your own from others' feelings. What doesn't belong to you belongs to someone else. Ask the Divine to clear that which isn't your own.

Beliefs

There are six primary types of beliefs:

Primary Belief	Negative Aspect	Positive Aspect
Worthiness	I am unworthy.	I am worthy.
Deserving	I don't deserve.	I do deserve.
Power	I am powerless.	I am powerful.
Value	I have no value	I am valuable.
Love	I am not lovable.	I am lovable.
Goodness	I am bad (or evil).	I am good.

You can arrive at any of these beliefs on your own. You can also take on others' beliefs and live them out. (Information on this process is available in *Advanced Chakra Healing*.) The key to sorting your own from others' beliefs is to center yourself in your heart and ask to intuitively know your own essential beliefs in regard to an issue. Any ideas or thoughts that don't align with this don't fit for you.

Illnesses and Diseases

To identify when you can take on another's illness or disease, center in the chakra with the presenting problem. Visual psychics should think of a presenting illness and ask it to form into an image. Now ask to see the source of this image. If it's not you, you'll know. Verbal psychics can ask to speak to the illness and demand that it honestly share its source. Kinesthetic psychics might first move into the state of the pure self and then imagine the illness dwelling as a contained energy within the first chakra. They can demand that a personal illness remain within the chakra, but that anything not of the pure self be expelled.

Patterns

You've likely absorbed someone else's pattern if one of the following rings true:

- You can't explain certain repetitive actions or behaviors with your own life story.
- No matter how hard you work on breaking a pattern, you can't.
- You feel like you are "under a spell," as if compelled into certain repetitive ways of being.
- You keep acting just like Mom or Dad, and you don't want to do so.

In the balance of this insert, I offer techniques and processes for energy work and energy mapping.

Five Steps for Safe Psychic Use

There's a five-step process for safely applying your psychic gifts to all energy work. I encourage you to use this process in all your Four Pathways undertakings.

1. *Ground and center.* Grounding involves anchoring your consciousness in a secure and trustworthy substance, such as the earth itself, a place of knowledge, a natural or spiritual force, or a spiritual quality. Centering involves locating your fully conscious self where you can access all your gifts and truths. You can center in a part of your body, an energy center, a concept, or a truth.
2. *Establish parameters.* Boundaries keep us inside of ourselves and keep what could harm us outside of ourselves. There are different forms of boundaries for each pathway. To establish the appropriate parameters for each pathway, use your key actions: intention on the elemental pathway, commanding on the power pathway, imagination on the imagination path-

way, and petitioning on the divine pathway.

3. *Conduct the goal*. When energy mapping, you will establish an objective and proceed toward it by following a list of tasks that has been laid out.
4. *Release energies*. In the course of achieving your goal, you may have freed energies that now need to be released. In the chapters on the four pathways, there are exercises for getting rid of energies that aren't your own, processing feelings, and doing any number of other tasks that might be necessary.
5. *Center, ground, and reestablish parameters*. Returning to your center is a way of returning to your everyday self. You can then ground in the appropriate energy and set parameters for everyday functioning.

Freeing Yourself from Others' Energies and Interference

Here are different ways to free yourself from energies that might be hampering you.

Reneging on Energy Contracts

Determining the nature of an energetic contract will help you choose the best method for removing it. To decipher a contract, respond to these questions:

- Am I one of the original creators of this contract, or was it created by something or someone else?
- If it wasn't me, how did I come to receive it? Is there something I must do, say, understand, or express to release myself from this contract?
- If I did enter this agreement, when did I do so? For what reason?

- What type of contract is this? An energetic cord? Life energy cord? A binding or an enigma? If one of the latter, who else is involved in or affected by this agreement?
- What is the nature of the contractual agreement? What am I giving? What am I receiving?
- How is this contract affecting me? The others around me or in the contract?
- What do I need to know to release myself from, to change, or to better use this contract? What feelings must I understand or express? What beliefs must I accept? What energy must I release or accept? (On the elemental pathway, ask these questions: What power levels must I free myself from? What power field must be brought to its optimum function?)
- What forgiveness or grace must I allow myself or the others involved?
- Am I now ready for this healing? If not, why not, and when will I be?

There are three main ways of exorcising energy contracts; these methods also work for hauntings or ancestral interference. They are different from cord or binding release in that they rely on your power to command and hold intention, rather than a healing process.

- *Rejection*. To reject a contract or interference, you must use 100 percent intention to refuse the contract and repel the energies attached to it. Might is right. If you command with more energy or intelligence than what's used against you, you will win. Request that all concerned receive divine healing from wounds remaining from eliminated contracts.
- *Containment*. You have the divine right to isolate yourself from negative sources. Simply command that the Divine immediately protect you. If you are mightier than your "foe," you can also demand the containment of any energies, forces, or entities that have been plaguing you.

- *Transformation*. By giving the energy of forgiveness, you are sending "white light" at the energy or entity that is bothering you. This energy offers grace to the interference or contract partners. If they accept the forgiveness, divine love offers healing, and they automatically release you. If they don't, the "white light" pushes them out of your boundaries and deals with them. Any energy that the other forces have been holding is automatically returned to you when you request transformation for all concerned.

The Transpersonal Process

If you think that you're dealing with assumed energies, you can conduct this ten-step, elemental pathway–based healing process:

1. Center yourself in the issue and ask the Divine to separate your own energies from any others'. Ask your own energy to step aside and wait awhile. You will communicate with it shortly.
2. Command that energies not your own create an image that can speak and communicate with you.
3. Demand that the energy now present itself in a representation that shows its truest form or nature.
4. Ask why this energy joined with you. What did it want to receive by this action? What did it receive? What did it take from you?
5. Now ask the energy of yourself, which has been separated out, what you received from joining with the other energy. What was your payoff? What did you expect to receive? What did you actually receive?
6. Ask yourself what you need to do, own, know, feel, learn, or experience to release the energy that is not your own.
7. Ask the other's energy what it needs to do, own, know, feel, learn, or experience to be willing to leave.

8. Release the energy that is not your own. If it doesn't want to go, ask for divine assistance. This is your right.
9. Cement your chakric and auric field back into place, first repairing any damage. Ask for divine assistance and healing now and as you integrate this change.
10. Commit to acting in a whole way for yourself.

Finding Your Fragments and Reclaiming Yourself

Not only do we implant others' energies, but we also give our own energy and parts of ourselves away. The following ten-step process works for recession and cordage to the self:

1. Ground and center.
2. Track the recessed energy to its location. You can look for cords, bindings, filaments, energy lines, and attachments; follow the flow of neutrons; or simply ask to see where the missing self or energies are at this time. If you are verbal, you can attune with your heartbeat and listen for the rhythm of the missing self in the universe.
3. Acknowledge the presence of the Divine in and around you for safety.
4. Psychically look at the situation. Are you caught or trapped? Willingly somewhere else? What aspect of the self is externalized and why? How is your life affected by the lack of this self, energy, or gifts?
5. What needs to occur to integrate this self or energy again? What do you need to know, understand, do, or learn? What does this self or energy need to know, understand, do, or learn?
6. When it and you are ready for integration, ask the Divine to bring the healing or release teams of angels on the scene, and other guardians of the Divine to assist. Allow this self or energy to be fully purified, cleansed, and transformed for integration, and ask that room be made inside of you

for it.

7. Ask the Divine to deal with energies that are not your own — whatever or whoever was holding the externalized self — and to completely sever and heal you from any energetic attachments.
8. As you allow integration, ask that you be told anything you must do to support a safe and easy incorporation.
9. Cement your chakric and auric fields back into place, first repairing any damage. Ask for Divine assistance and healing now and as you integrate this change.
10. Commit to acting in a whole way for yourself.

Energetic Cleansing with Physical Properties

Repairing after an energetic release can take some time. Here are some elemental pathway–based measures that can speed the process, aid in recovery after possession and integration work, and take care of cleansing from others' energies on a daily basis:

- *White wash:* Picture the Divine's white energy flooding your body as if through a fountain, flowing from above, through your body, then down through your tenth chakra. Ask that the earth, which will recycle them, transmute all energies.
- *Black tea bath:* Boil five to six black tea bags in one gallon of water over high heat for ten minutes. Remove the teabags and add the liquid only to your bath. Set the intention of flushing feelings and toxins that are not useful. When done, add colloidal oatmeal to the bath or use baking soda on your skin to restore your skin's pH.
- *Implements:* Select a rock, amulet, or other tool. With intention, use it to absorb others' energies. Cleanse weekly in the rain, in Epsom salts and water, or through intention.
- *Shaman techniques:* Use candles, incense, drumming, or burning sage to cleanse yourself or your home of others' energies.

Moving through Time for Information and Healing

By moving backward, sideways, and forward in time, you can figure out the causes of various problems and find solutions. Here are three basic techniques.

Regressing Regressions involve looking back into the past or relinking with a part of you that is stuck in the past, in order to gather data regarding a current problem. You can also potentially use regression to free yourself from the past and to change the past so that the present can be different.

Caution: For serious or scary issues, I suggest that you work with a professional to conduct a regression. Certified hypnotherapists are trained to work with the issues and feelings that arise, as are licensed psychologists who use Eye Movement Desensitization and Reprocessing (EMDR), a particularly helpful form of regression. For lighter issues, here is a five-step process that you can use.

Regression Exercise

1. Prepare. Ground and center. Think of your causal issue. After asking for Divine protection and guidance, ask which chakra is key to this causal issue. Now open your psychic senses by asking the Divine to fully open your chakras and to allow only loving use of your gifts.
2. Enter. Sense or see the chakra center causal to your issue. There you will spot a door, mirror, or opening of some sort. Ask the Divine to guide you through this portal and into the situation that created your current predicament.
3. Research and clarify. Once in the situation, ask to see, hear, know, and experience everything necessary to obtain the information or healing that you need. State that your conscious self will remember all that you are experiencing. Then ask to understand what decisions you (or someone else) made during this time period that still affect you today. Now ask for

clarification. Why did you make these decisions? What other choices were available? What did you need to learn? What do you still need to learn?

4. Heal. Ask the Divine to tell you what healing and forgiveness are necessary. Is it appropriate to change the circumstances of that time? How are you to do so? If you are to leave the situation status quo, ask what wisdom will enable you to leave the past in the past. Now, ask the Divine to help you make any necessary changes in the prior time period. Accept the healing energies.
5. Return and infuse. Ask the Divine if it is appropriate to bring any changes forward so as to affect the present. Is it more helpful to simply make changes in the present, and if so, which ones? Remain in the situation until you feel complete and whole with what happened and who you were at that time. Now request the Divine to return you to the present and to bring with you the learning, energy, wisdom, and information you need to make today a better place. Ask the Divine to help you internalize all appropriate learning or healing through all of your levels in a way that will be safe and easy. Establish any new boundaries for your now-changed self. Ground and center, and return fully to the present. Ask the Divine for additional protection and guidance as you integrate this information and infuse the past into the present.

Projecting

Projecting is a form of shamanic journeying. When journeying, mystics send an aspect of themselves or their consciousness in search of wisdom, data, or healing energies.

Journeying can take you near or far, into the past, present, or future, but it isn't always easy to do without guidance. I use the term *projecting* to describe journeying into only the present time.

On the divine pathway, healing occurs through expansion. Projecting is an elemental pathway–based means of expanding into the corners of reality that might hold data or healing that you need. Here is a five-step process for using projection for healing purposes:

Projecting Exercise

1. Prepare. Using the steps of grounding, centering, and protecting, ask the Divine to connect you fully with your spirit-self. Breathe deeply and imagine that you are fully invested in your spirit, which is inside of your body and also able to expand fully around you. Encompass your body in your own spirit and then "feel out to the edges."
2. Travel. Sense the presence of your spirit, which continues to envelop your body, as it swells into the room and then outdoors. Notice that nothing hurts you; everything simply is what it is. Your spirit is inviolate and remains its own pure self no matter what it touches or surrounds. Now think of your causal issue. Simply expand your consciousness as your spirit enters a place or space that contains everything you've yet to learn about this issue. Perhaps you're someplace three-dimensional, perhaps you're in the Netherlands, or perhaps you're in heaven. You have now journeyed to exactly where you need to be, without leaving your body behind.
3. Learn. What learning has been awaiting you in this spacetime? What wisdom is yours to acknowledge and to grasp? Why is it important to understand this information, in reference to the "you" of the "current time"?
4. Embrace. Fully embrace both this spacetime and the learning that you came to learn. Know that you are really embracing yourself.
5. Infuse and return. As quickly as possible, infuse the learning and the spirit-self of the visited spacetime through the energy field connecting the body-based self with the travel-

ing self. As you accept the learning into the here and now, decide to live fully in this body, in this time, with the energies of truth. Ask the Divine to help you internalize all appropriate learning or healing through all of your levels in a way that will be safe and easy. Establish any new boundaries for your now-changed self. Ground and center, and return fully to the present. Ask the Divine for additional protection and guidance as needed, until you are fully integrated.

Futuring

The future is really a net of possibilities that surround your current self. You don't have to "go anywhere" to access the future. The lines of the future are being drawn around you as you sit and read this book!

Here is a five-step process for futuring:

Futuring Exercise

1. Prepare. When futuring, first ground, center, and resonate with your spirit-self. Then attune with the energies of the future that are around you already. You'll see that it's like being surrounded by a grid of Christmas lights! These are magnetic, proton-based timelines that link to possible futures. What do you desire to see? What is your goal? Look around at all the twinkling opportunities and times that respond to your question. What is the most likely path? The best path? Ask the Divine to assure you of your choice, as you prepare for "liftoff."
2. "Travel." Ask the Divine to show which line your spirit would follow if it weren't affected by anything adverse or unhealthy. Know that futuring doesn't actually entail any traveling. Instead of sending your consciousness into the future, pull the lighted line as if you are fishing. Reel it to the front side of your heart and ask to perceive it with True Vision — the vision of your own spirit.

3. Learn. What do you perceive? Ask the Divine to guide you to respond to the imaging pulled from the future. Are you to learn from it? Own it? Magnetize this potential so it occurs, or do the opposite?
4. Embrace or heal. Can you accept the learning and healing from the future or the future self? If affirmative, assume a position of gratitude for the knowledge or healing received, and allow the future web to shape around you. Embrace the future in the here and now.
5. Infuse and integrate. Close your eyes and connect again with your body. Ground, center, and resonate with the decisions that you have made. Ask the Divine to help you continue to integrate your choices safely and with love toward yourself and others.

Healing Feelings

Not all feelings are assumed from others. Here is a high-level spiritual exercise to heal feelings of your own that might underpin an issue.

1. Select an issue or a problem. Accept the discomfort it is causing in your life and in your body. Don't resist. You might still actually feel the discomfort in your system, such as still needing to vomit if you have the flu.
2. Know that this discomfort does not exist in every aspect of yourself. There are different versions of the same reality. There is a place where you have illness, issues, a problem, or a need, and a space in which your needs are fulfilled in a way that makes the problems unnecessary. If there is discomfort inside of you, there is also a space of comfort.
3. Breathe deeply and associate with this state of comfort. A visual psychic may picture the discomfort as a form apart from the body. A kinesthetic intuitive will have to feel the discomfort and move through it until finding a place of clearness in the body. A verbal psychic will command him-

or herself to a comfortable space. You can say that you want to be in your "place of purity" or the "state of comfort." If none of these methods works, ask for divine help. You simply want your consciousness placed in the state of comfort.

4. Now the critical element: feel the feeling connecting you to the discomfort. And I mean feeling as in part of an emotion, not the emotion itself. A discomfort is always energetically composed of a variety of feelings, beliefs, energies, and even entities and forces. This aggregate connects with you because at some moment in time you had a feeling about what was going on. Get back to your original feeling.
5. Keep feeling. If another feeling arises, stay with it or consider getting a friend or therapist to help you go to the core feeling.
6. Accept your awareness about the feeling and ask yourself why you had this feeling. This feeling arose historically because of a perceived need. What was it? What need is this feeling pointing out?
7. Petition to feel the Divine's acceptance of your need. *Look for patterns, strongholds, illnesses, or issues that stem from a need that you believe has not been met.* The need has not been met because you judged it, not because the Divine judged it. When we judge a need, we freeze the feeling about the need, and then we go about creating backward and distorted ways to get our need met.
8. Petition for the Divine to meet the original need.
9. Know that you can now complete your relationship with the original feeling. This knowledge will open to an even deeper level of truth and eventually give way to a spiritual feeling. The spiritual feeling will generate through the superluminal body, activating the spiritual genetics and changing the conditions in your body. Your *spiritual genetics* are described in chapter 7. For now, know that they are basically your ideal genetics, as prescribed by your spirit.

10. Accept the learning. It will change you.

Forgiveness

Forgiveness is a gift to the self. The word *forgiveness* means the act of "for giving." Which energies are meant to be given to someone else and which are to be kept to yourself? Which energies were supposed to be kept by someone else and which are to be given to you?

Forgiveness Exercise Here is a forgiveness exercise that invites spiritual healing.

1. Invoke the Divine's energy of grace, which is power in love.
2. Center and ask the Divine to help you generate the actual substance of grace outward, from your center to all other aspects of your self.
3. Petition the Divine to grant grace to anything and anyone who has harmed you or continues to negatively affect you. Ask the same for yourself.
4. Offer choices. The conscious direction of grace offers three choices to all individuals, entities, and consciousnesses currently preying on you: to transform, to leave, or to receive consequences. Regardless of what choice another being makes, you can make one that is self-loving and self-respecting, which will involve freeing the others' energies from you. If at first an energy or entity doesn't leave when invited to do so, either contain or rebuke it, handing it over to its higher self or to the Divine.
5. Completion. Invite the Divine to complete the healing by returning your own energies to you, establishing the correct parameters for your renewed integration, and blessing the other people or beings.

Steps to Energy Mapping

You can produce an energy map for each pathway or select one pathway to begin your healing. Generally, the same steps are involved in energy mapping any of the pathways. I will share an example of energy mapping on the elemental pathway, because it is the most complicated of the Four Pathways.

There are two parts to the energy mapping process: diagnosis and healing. Here are the steps:

Part One: Diagnostic Steps

1. Get paper and pen or prepare some other way to remember the information you will be receiving. You will be energy mapping pictorially, drawing or making other notes to record what you learn in these diagnostic steps. Visual psychics can simply sketch what they see. If you receive verbal or tonal information, write down descriptions of what you hear and in which chakras. The same applies for kinesthetic information; describe the types of feelings you receive in answer to different questions.
2. Ground and center.
3. Establish parameters.
4. Select a starting chakra. Refer to the chart of the various types of cancers and their partnered chakras, or trust your intuition to figure out your baseline chakra. In the case of cancer, you want to start with the chakra related to the primary cancer site. If there isn't one, select either the first chakra for serious cases or the seventh to read for the Divine's interpretation of the cancer.
5. Access your strongest psychic chakra or the one that's most logical to use to energy map.
6. You will now examine the primary chakra for diagnostic issues according to your selected pathway. The particular questions you should ask on specific pathways are listed in

the chapters about these pathways. Generic issues to examine for include the following:

- Type of cancer charge: negative, positive, or neutral.
- Spin of the cancer.
- Spin of the chakra's inner and outer wheels.
- Coloration of the cancer versus the rest of the chakra.
- Tone of the cancer versus the rest of the chakra.
- Symbology of the cancer and symbols in the rest of the chakra.
- Location of interference and connections to other places.
- Connections of the cancer to other chakras; for instance, check to see if there are cords connecting the cancerous state to other chakras or energies in the body.
- Connections of the cancer to other aspects of the self, such as spirit, soul, mind, heart, and body.

7. Record your answers on your paper or diagram. After illustrating your responses, examine your findings and go deeper intuitively. Now write the responses you receive when considering each of the following:

    - Reason for the cancer, as related to the type of cancer. For instance, with negatively charged cancers you will look for emotional, physical, or psychic causes as well as issues with power; with positively charged cancers, spiritual beliefs and fears; with neutral cancers, needs for love.
    - Timing of the cancer. When did this cancer begin? Know that you can look to prior existences and prebirth, as well as this lifetime.
    - Source of the cancer. Did the cancer begin inside of you or with something or someone else?
    - Percentage of the cancer caused by self versus interference, such as curses, bindings, cords, hauntings, or assumption of others' energies and feelings.

- Vibration of your harmonic. Cancers are out of tune with your core harmonic. What is your core harmonic?
- Vibration of the chakra. What is the correct vibration of your chakra that is the primary site?
- Vibration of the master cancer cells. What frequencies are they holding or not? How is that affecting the surrounding cells and organs?
- What is holding the cancer in place? What is the data instructing the cancer to stay in your body? Is there an issue within the chakra keeping the cancer within your body?
- Are there sources, such as energies or beings, either inside or outside of you keeping this cancer locked into place?
- Information from your subconscious. What is the message your inner self is trying to give you by giving you cancer?
- Information from your spirit. What need might you really be trying to meet, as informed by your spirit and the Divine's spirit?

8. Create a statement of need that summarizes your conclusions in a few sentences.

Part Two: Healing Steps

After creating an energy map and an understanding of what initiated the cancer, review your work, paying special attention to your statement of need. You will now prepare a plan of action, considering the following issues — again, more specifically on each pathway.

- Overall need.
- Help that you can draw upon, both visible and invisible.
- Spins that will meet the need.
- Colors that will meet the need.
- Tones that will meet the need.

- Symbology that will meet the need.
- Interference and connections to release.
- Connections to make externally.
- Connections to make internally.
- Connections to make to other aspects of the self.
- Reasons to release the cancer.
- Ways to meet the need differently through behavior, emotional expression, attitude and thinking, spiritual understandings, relationship connections, or psychic activity.

- Ways to release the "self" at the age at which the cancer was developed or the reasons for it were conducted.
- Ways to release energies (beings, energies, consciousness, cords, and the like) causing or enforcing the cancer; ways to forgive others and the self for this occurrence.
- Ways to heal the cancer at its source. Will this involve moving to a different pathway?
- Ways to change the vibration of cancer, chakra, body, or aspect of self. Will this involve shifting to a new pathway to make the job easier?
- Ways to permanently alter the master cancer cells. Will this take a shift to a different pathway?
- Ways to assume the beliefs that will bring forth the whole self. Will this take a pathway shift?

Linking the Pathways: A Means of Moving Energies between Pathways

You link pathways through assuming your wholeness. Here is an exercise that will help.

Transferring Energy on the Pathways

The real link between you and all pathways is through your spiritual essence or whole self. Automatically, energy and change are transferred through all the pathways. You can also consciously control this process through this exercise.

1. Select a chakra as a focus. This can be the chakra you've been working on for healing or any favorite chakra. Now figure out which pathway you're currently standing on, or select one as a starting point.
2. The center of this chakra serves as an elevator shaft to all other chakras on all other pathways. You can do one of two things through this elevator:

- Deliver information or energies to other pathways
- Obtain information or energies from other pathways

3. Decide what you want to accomplish and then proceed.
4. Allow full integration on all pathways and inside of yourself.

PART *Two*

chapter six

Energy Mapping on the Elemental Pathway

Just you remember, it's not what things look like that matters. It's what's inside. *The* art *of it.*

—Joanne Harris, *Blackberry Wine*[1]

Travel the elemental pathway under these conditions:

- You are already taking physical action to prevent or battle cancer.
- You know you need to change your beliefs or attitudes to heal from cancer.
- You think you have to deal differently with feelings to heal from cancer.
- You are willing to make behavioral changes to heal from cancer.
- You are a "here and now" person.
- You want to use the elemental pathway as a basis, then supplement your care with one of the other pathways.
- You most often rely on your first, second, third, or tenth chakras.

The Elemental Pathway: The Basic Units of Life

I once had a holistic practitioner show me the medley of supplements he used in his practice.

"Pick your poison," he said.

I laughed and asked him why he considered his "cures" poisonous.

"There's been nothing invented that fixes all people, all of the time," he said. "What's good for one is bad for the other. It's what inside the person that makes something work or not."

To find what's poison or cure for *you*, you must get to the particulars of the elemental pathway.

The elemental pathway is the most basic pathway. This is the "particle universe." Healing on this pathway is always about particles and particulars. This search for underlying causes is part of a reductionistic healing process.

Reductionism involves analyzing something down to its simplest elements or most primary organizing system. The goal is to understand what's at the root of an issue or problem. Then, if necessary, you can start with new building blocks, an altered set of elements, or a brand new system to meet the goal of creating health rather than disease.

You begin a reductionistic process by looking for patterns. If you can perceive a pattern holding a disease in place, you can outline its components. When you have cancer you examine for *cancer-producing patterns* — those patterns that establish the conditions for cancer. To get underneath the surface of a pattern, you test for variables to see which ones are supporting a disease, which ones are useful, and which might be neutral. Once you figure out the unhealthy parts of a pattern, you can "break the pattern" in one of several ways:

- Eliminate the disease-producing part of the pattern
- Discard the entire pattern

- Establish new behaviors or patterns, in part or entirely

At heart, both traditional and holistic medicine works the same way as I've outlined. Although these disciplines don't use the term *cancer-producing patterns*, both look for these phenomena to prevent, diagnose, or attempt to heal cancer.

Cancer and the Elemental Pathway

As I've noted, the elemental pathway encompasses mainstream and holistic philosophies and care, but it approaches them in a different light. When using these healing efforts on the elemental pathway, you:

- Assume wholeness rather than brokenness
- Allow yourself to bring this wholeness to the surface through the various activities that you undertake to heal from cancer
- Invite a two-way transfer of energy, as your elemental pathway work is translated to all other pathways, and energies from other pathways are automatically sent to the elemental pathway; this is done through your whole self, which unifies all four pathways

Let's look at ways to accomplish all three goals.

Tools and Healing on the Elemental Pathway

Healing cancer on this pathway includes these components:

- Using Intention to Surface Wholeness
- Energies on the Elemental Pathway
- Healing on the Physical: The Basis of Elemental Healing

- Basic Energy Healing: Special Elemental Techniques
- Helpers on the Elemental Pathway

Using Intention to Surface Wholeness

The chief way to make elemental changes is through intention. An *intention* is a quality or state of mind formed around a purpose. When you intend to do something, everything in your body, mind, and soul works together to make it happen. To make things happen on the elemental pathway, you must focus full intention on your goals.

I once met Baba Sri Shiva, the master who taught Dr. Wayne Dyer how to manifest. I heartily enjoyed one of the exercises, which was to chant the following around an objective: "I must, I must, I must get what I want. I will not stop until I get what I want." Dedication such as this activates your first and second chakra energies to full vitality, thus fueling you with the life energy needed to defeat cancer. It also activates the manifesting side of healing. If you can think "manifesting" instead of "healing," you'll invite your body to assume wholeness instead of brokenness.

Energies on the Elemental Pathway

This section discusses the energy bodies and basic energetic healing principles of the elemental pathway. There are many energy bodies on the elemental pathway; they are called the *managing energy bodies* and the *secondary energy bodies.* Each regulates a physical, emotional, mental, and spiritual set of concerns, in addition to playing relational and psychic roles.

You'll find a complete list of the many elemental energy bodies available for healing in *Advanced Chakra Healing*; here I will present only a few before moving right into showing you how to apply this knowledge for healing through traditional as well as energetic means. It's important to know that you don't have to throw out the basics of physical care, such as surgery, diet, and exercise; rather, you can supplement your work with chakra-based techniques.

In general, when you work elementally you should start with your primary cancer chakra, which is usually the chakra relating to the primary cancer site. Address the cause, and you may resolve the problem.

The Chakras On the elemental pathway, a change made within a chakra is also transferred to all other areas of concern regulated by that chakra, as well as to other chakras on this and other pathways.

The Spiritual Points There are twenty of these higher chakra points in your broader energy field. These channel spiritual truths into your body and serve as elevator shafts between the elemental and divine pathways. They also connect directly into your vertebrae. You can learn more about how to use them in *Advanced Chakra Healing: Energy Mapping* and *New Chakra Healing.*

The Auric Fields These bands of light provide structure, screening, and protection. Paired with the chakras, each auric band is responsible for communicating that chakra's needs to the world and for attracting energies to meet these needs. If you have cancer, the auric bands related to those chakras are not functioning properly. You must assess these bands and clear up problems to enable the overall auric field to better protect you.

The Morphogenetic Fields Perceived through the tenth auric field, these fields are highly important for diagnosing sources of ancestral or soul-inherited issues, as well as those from society. You can read the physical and energetic programs for genetic cancers; cancers caused by environmental issues (such as toxic food, water, or chemicals) and geophysical disturbances; cancers created through ancestral curses, hauntings, or inherited auric field weaknesses; and any number of other issues. Treat such cancers in the originating chakra, and translate the changes throughout all auric fields or via the etheric mirror. (The latter is described in this section as well as in the chapter 5 insert and chapter 8.)

The Energy Egg The inner layer of this egg most closely identifies with the elemental pathway. One of the easiest ways to examine this inner layer is through the pineal gland, which reads consciousness. Center yourself in this organ, which is in the lower part of your brain, almost in between your eyes. You will detect white, gray, or black energies and sometimes red. Concentrate on energies that don't match the general background of your chakra or the coloration of the energy egg's inner layer. These are the energies causing cancer. Blue or off-black cancers are negative, off-white or yellow ones are positive, and red tones indicate neutral-based cancers. You can remain within the pineal gland and energy map from here, as well as conduct your healing changes.

You can also psychically peruse this energy egg to pinpoint the exact causes of your cancer. For healing purposes, you can journey within the inner layer of the egg to picture healing choices and your healing potential. Through the third layer, you can access spiritual waves or powerful spiritual energies that can correct the cancer. (Chapter 9 describes this divine pathway process.) The second layer is best used in tandem with your imagination on the imagination pathway to see your healing and life choices. You can, however, access all of the energy egg layers through the elemental pathway.

The Etheric Mirror The etheric mirror, or Christ body, contains the ideal "programming" for your physical body. This programming supports your spiritual purpose and life plan. Use cording in a positive way to establish links of white light between the primary or secondary cancer sites and the same areas in the etheric mirror. Set up a spin from the etheric mirror so you transfer energy from this body back into the physical body. If necessary, ask for spiritual helpers to guide your process and keep it going. Transferring energy from the etheric mirror to the physical body is an ideal way to reprogram your DNA, using your own ideal coding.

The Akashic Records Although technically not an energy body, this collection of information holds vibration and forms its own "organ," which feeds information from the past into your soul, mind, and body. A recording of all information pertinent to you, the Akashic Records are accessible through every chakra, but they are most easily accessed through your eighth chakra. On the elemental pathway, obtain these records by centering in your eighth chakra. Now psychically perceive your Akashic Records. Request divine guidance to turn to the page that relates the cause of your cancer. If needed, ask the Divine to bring you back into the experience of this cancer's origins and conduct your healing from there.

The records can also identify cures or healing processes. Connect with your Records and ask to perceive the pages highlighting potential cures in the past, present, or future.

The Shadow Records The Shadow Records are, well, a mere shadow away from the parenting Akashic Records! Although the Akashic Records reflect "reality," the Shadow Records store everything that you could have become.

Many illnesses are caused by regret — the perception that we've lost our chance to love or succeed. If your cancer is negative or negatively charged, it might involve feelings and beliefs repressed through regret. To find out, journey into your eighth chakra and think about the cancer. Don't psychically link with the cancer; instead sense the energy that hovers around the cancer site. This energy is the shadow of your cancer. Ask the Divine or your spiritual guides to help you energy map the shadow reality. For healing, work with the Forgiveness Exercise given in the insert or the exercise "Reading the Book of Life for a Cancer-Free Life" in chapter 7.

The realm of the Shadow shows not only what didn't become, but also what could become. You can also use the Shadow Records to make treatment decisions. Think of a potential treatment modality and then look into the shadow area around the cancer to see how this therapy affects the cancer. You'll note if the cancer grows, shrinks, or disappears while viewing the Shadow Records. But don't ignore logic and professional input; talk over any treatment alternatives with your physician.

The Physical Body Yes, this is an elemental pathway energy body! Your physical self is made of information-energy, just as your etheric energy bodies are. This is why I'm going to provide a lot of information about physical treatments of cancer in this chapter.

Healing on the Physical: The Basis of Elemental Healing

The elemental pathway is essentially physical, as are current cancer treatments. The main difference between working purely physically and working the physical on the elemental pathway is that when care is provided in and through a chakra, the gain is transferred throughout your entire system, and you open to healing energies from the Greater Reality. With this in mind, I offer a few suggestions on how to open traditional or complementary care to pathway strengths.

Enhancing Typical Traditional Treatments for Cancer

Standard treatment usually involves surgery, chemotherapy, radiation, and biological therapy. Medicines and drugs are often given in an attempt to control carcinogenic factors, such as estrogen levels in women. Here are elemental pathway approaches to support the three most common traditional treatments.

Surgery Work with a holistic provider or nutritionist to plan a dietary and supplemental protocol for pre- and postsurgery. Run all choices by your primary physician, as some supplements and herbs — such as aspirin and vitamin E — cause problems with clotting. In general, consider upping your protein, as amino acids are building blocks for recovery.

Do anything possible to go into surgery with a calm attitude. Work with a massage therapist and listen to music. Use pink and gold when meditating, as these colors are vibrationally the best choices for physical healing. Use the exercises for particular concerns provided in the chapter 5 insert. I recommend the Transpersonal Process for preparing the organ or body area to release tissue and cancer easily and the Forgiveness Exercise for going into surgery with a clean heart. Set your power fields most affected by the surgery at their highest frequency, which will aid in recovery.

Right before surgery, expand pink through your auric field and envision it in the operating room, with the intention of having the Divine hold you and everyone in the surgical room in divine love. Check to see if music is played in the operating room; if so, choose your own selection. Line up people to pray or meditate for you during surgery. Post your spiritual guides at all four corners of the room during surgery.

There are several postsurgical stages. Initially, you will need pain relief and to follow your doctor's plan. At some point, it will be beneficial to review your diet and supplement protocol.

Anesthesia and medications such as antibiotics greatly inhibit your immune system and alter your pH balance. Review a recovery diet with a professional and consider detoxification when you have recovered from surgery. Detoxification usually involves taking antioxidants and using acidophilus or eating yogurt. Support your immune system by considering supplements such as shiitake mushrooms or olive leaf extract. Yeast and fungus infections often develop after surgery; these can sometimes be deterred with the acidophilus or cleansers like wild oregano extract; mineral and vitamin supplementation in addition to your antioxidant regime; a diet low in sugar, milk, gluten, and yeast; and green tea in place of coffee, as green tea has been shown to be a powerful antioxidant with cancer-fighting properties. You can maximize the results of nutrients and supplements by imaging these substances affecting the spin in your chakra, adding spiritual energetic forces as described on the power pathway, and working with your spiritual helpers to increase their effectiveness, as described in the "Helpers on the Elemental Pathway" section of this chapter.

Remember as well a basic lesson from physics: two materials never actually "touch"; there is always infinite space between two objects, even if they seem to come into contact. At the quanta level, your tissues were never cut by surgical equipment! Image the space around your wound area as open and pure, and fill this space with energies, harmonics, tones, or thoughts healing to you. Select colors or energies that are ultraviolet or pale blue and therefore anti-inflammatory.

Chemotherapy and Radiation The drugs and chemicals used in chemotherapy are poisonous, as is radiation — as they should be, to kill cancer cells! However, both processes are also toxic to your healthy cells.

Work with a holistic practitioner such as naturopath or nutritionist to select a nutritional and supplement protocol. You need different properties during chemotherapy and radiation than you do after your treatment course, as you don't want to cancel out the "good work" of your treatment. Refer to the exercises under the food section in this chapter to amplify or decrease the effects of compounds and elements. You want to amp up your nutritional and supplement value at all times. You also want to maximize the potency of your treatments during and immediately after them; then, when it's time to detoxify, you should decrease the energy of these poisonous substances.

Remember the discussion of receptor cells and feelings in chapter 3? If you have cancer, chances are the receptors on the cells in the physical area and surrounding it are full of neuropeptides dangerous to your health. Surgery brings benefits, as it involves the removal of these cells. Chemotherapy and radiation aim at killing these cells, but the neuropeptides occupy the receptor sites that the poisons could plug into. Healthy cells, on the other hand, have vulnerable receptor cells. It always pays to deal with your emotional issues before and during treatment, and also to image your cells' release of the cancer-stimulating neuropeptides before and after treatment. You want the malignant cells susceptible to the poison.

As well, direct positive thoughts and feelings at your healthy cells. Picture your hypothalamus producing neuropeptides that are attuned with your personal harmonic and "ask" your thalamus, which structures cells, to reorganize your tissues into healthy shapes. In place of the five core feelings, select truths like faith, love, healing, and joy. The energy of faith will stimulate the production of neuropeptides that culminate in advanced healing properties in your body.

Before and during treatment, refer to this chapter's section on elements and consider using stone or earth to wall off healthy tissue, so the chemotherapy and radiation affect only the cancer cells. Consider placing an energy marker (as described in the chapter 5 insert) on the tumor site or over the cancer cells, and then image this same marker on the incoming poisons. You might want to envision an "x" as a marker, imaging this symbol on the tumor and the chemicals. You can also select a tone, preferably an aberrant or flat one, and psychically vibrate the cancer site and the chemical medicines at that rate. Kinesthetics can sense the disconcerting nature of the cancer and feel this same discord when receiving chemotherapy. Ask the Divine to attach that negative sensation only to malignant cells and the medicine. These matching markers will attract the two forces to each other, leaving your healthy cells in peace. If you are working the power pathway, consider attaching a powerful generative spiritual force to the incoming energies, so they carry a real "blast."

If you are familiar with the power pathway, also consider inserting a degenerative spiritual force around the tumor site, setting its spin so as to spin away any toxic fields or dead cells. If you're not working the power pathway simultaneously, work with spin. Make sure to set the inner wheel of your primary cancer chakra in reverse so it can spin the toxins out of your body. Also set the eighth chakra's inner wheel in reverse, as well as the eighth auric field, to cleanse your body. Check too that you have a positive spin on your lymph system and nodes, so they can carry out toxins generated by the standard treatments. You can use generative or degenerative spiritual forces from the power pathway to amplify any of these procedures.

After standard treatment, it's even more important to magnify the effectiveness of products used for detoxification and to generate helpful energy for your healthy cells. Also maximize any posttreatment drugs, such as those taken for long-term breast cancer prevention, using the techniques already described.

Representative List of Holistic Cancer Treatments Alternative treatments include adjunctive psychological approaches, such as psychotherapy, imagery, group therapy, and cancer support groups; macrobiotics; nutritional-metabolic programs, including various diets, supplements, and herbal treatments; traditional Chinese medicine; religious, energetic, psychic, and spiritual healing; technological treatments, such as the use of computers, light frequencies, and vibrational technologies; electromagnetic therapies; homeopathy and other vibrational medicines; manipulative treatments, such as chiropractic and massage; folk and shamanic treatments; and unconventional cancer therapies, including laetrile, Hoxley herbs, psychoimmunology, or immunosupportive therapies.

Many holistic treatments are described throughout this chapter. As well, consider using some of the techniques covered in the previous section, "Chemotherapy and Radiation," as addenda to holistic care — specifically, adding extra energies to supplements, nutritional foods, and water; eliminating negative energies from the body; and using power pathway forces to bolster life-enhancing substances and reduce cancer materials.

Through the Chakras: Body-Based Healing Your chakras are key to helping you decide which changes in behavior and lifestyle can best support your full recovery from cancer. There are several practical ways you can negotiate healing, none of which take much money. These involve meeting your basic needs from assumed wholeness, which requires treating yourself as if you love yourself fully.

The rest of the techniques in this section work the elemental pathway and the chakras for cancer-free life.

Basic Life Needs and the Chakras

Basic needs are regulated by particular chakras.

- Shelter: Tenth (environment) and first (clothing)
- Breathing: Tenth (environment) and fourth (lungs)
- Water: First (skin), fifth (drinking), and all other in-body chakras
- Touch: First (skin and genital entry points) and fifth (eating)
- Movement: All
- Food: All

Shelter That Sustains Your tenth chakra monitors your relationship with nature and the environment. Your home can be programmed to be a sacred site for healing and support your healing around the clock.

Use your psychic perception to center in your tenth chakra and then think of one of the following:

- Plants, trees, and flowers
- Fountains or even bowls of water
- Stones, rocks, and crystals
- Colors, fabrics, and textures
- Music and sounds

Picture, sense, or listen for guidance. What items carry energies that could help you? Will anything you currently own bolster your healing? Do you need to buy or borrow something that will? Once you establish this item in your home, ask the Divine to open your tenth chakra to the beneficial healing properties it carries. You might picture a line of white light flowing from the object to you.

Remember to consider rooms you spend considerable time in. If you are affected by interference, consider using oil or sage smoke to mark the windowsills and doorways with the symbol of a cross within a circle. This symbol seals your home against potentially harmful energies.

Regarding clothing, remember that color, fabric, and metals are made of energy. Center in your first chakra and think of various colors and clothing items. What colors boost your health? Picture the cancer cells. Are there any clothing items that seem to reduce their potency? Consider your jewelry or belt buckles. Silver is a conduit and enables information gathering. Gold commands physical healing. Copper helps cleanse the blood, and platinum increases spiritual awareness. Think of all components of dress to support your healing.

The Power of Breath Your fourth chakra is charged with taking in and releasing air, a powerful element for healing. Detoxification is magnified when the lungs conduct their job in rhythm with the tenth chakra. Your energy system pulses toxins into the earth through the tenth chakra and accesses earth energy from the tenth chakra to empower your breathing.

Some cancers are related to environmental sensitivities carried on the air, including chemical toxicity from glues, paint, carpets, pesticides, secondary smoke, air emissions, power lines, and more. Even if bad air isn't the specific cause of your cancer, it certainly isn't helping you. You must cleanse your body through your breath for effective detoxification. Consider getting an air purifier or ion machine.

Rhythmic breathing performs a vital spiritual function. The word for *spirit* is the same as the word for *breath* in Greek, Hebrew, and Latin. The element of air carries information that is spiritual. By breathing deeply, you accept spiritual information that can heal. By exhaling completely, you release the old ideas and poisons keeping you from getting well. Do this type of breathing with intention for extra potency.

Cleansing through Water Your body is over 75 percent water. Water is the single most important healing substance. Elementally composed of a crystalline structure, it can be programmed to carry helpful messages that are life changing.
Consider the work of Dr. M. Emoto of Japan, a physicist who has taken pictures of water that holds energy. The cells of the water alter shape in response to different ideas. In my work as co-owner of a Minneapolis-based energy clinic, my associate — a biomedical inventor — and I program water for healing purposes. We've seen significant results when this water is applied for change.

Water molecules hold powerful spiritual forces within them. Consider the use of water for baptism. This simple physical substance when infused with spiritual intention unlocks vital forces of change. I believe that water carries a truth that stimulates heart enzymes for love, which in turn alters the hormone programs of the adrenals and the pineal gland, thereby establishing connections with your spiritual genetics, your personal harmonic, and the Divine. This truth enables healing in your body as well as manifestation of spiritual desires.

You can program drinking water for healing purposes with intention. The most simple method is to pray over the water, then lock in the changes with symbols printed at the bottom of the glass; a cross with a circle always works.

Awakening through Touch Touch primarily affects the first auric field and chakra, also generating energy for healing throughout your entire system. Studies show that babies who aren't touched will sicken or die, even if their other primary needs are met.

Touch passes energy. There is bad touch, as with sexual or physical abuse. I've had a client heal from cancer by ridding herself of the energy of sexual abuse, with no other type of treatment. Good touch heals. If you don't have someone who can hug or touch you, use other first chakra modes. Get a massage. Sleep with a baby blanket or a soft stuffed animal. Use infrared blankets and material, which promote healing.

Moving Out Cancer through Movement Exercise causes energetic responses in the body. Movement alters the spin of the energy organs, physical organs, and individual cells. Here are examples of specific activities as they pertain to healing from cancer.

- *Walking:* Excellent for cancers in all chakras. Walking opens every chakra and creates a flow of energy between them.
- *Running:* Speeds up all chakras to work uniformly toward desired goals. Set the goal of cleansing yourself from toxins, gaining ground on the cancer, or becoming free of disease.
- *Biking:* Ideal for chakras one and ten, this lower-body exercise opens you to earth energy for moving forward.
- *Swimming:* Swimming sustains you during stress and allows full integration of spiritual energies in your spine. To infuse

yourself with good energy, focus your thoughts on the spiritual points as you swim.

- *Tennis and racquetball:* Are useful for working through relationship-based strongholds causing cancer.
- *Downhill skiing:* Ensures flow under adversity.
- *Weightlifting:* Empowers you for hard times and strengthens your healthy cells.
- *Yoga:* Enhances kundalini flow. Do yoga while inserting spiritual energetics into the DNA of abnormal cells.
- *Martial arts:* Increases life energy and connects spiritual energies with physical strengths. Establish a discipline of higher chakras and the higher self over lower chakras and the lower self.
- *Dancing:* Expresses your spirit through your body.

Fueling Life through Food Besides water, food is the most important healing substance you can use physically. When combined with chakra healing, food takes on medicinal value.

There are dozens of factors to consider when managing food to achieve health. A few include pH balance, metabolic disruptors and assistants, the role of the elements, and foods for primary chakra sites. After considering these four areas, we'll examine the complex arena of diet supplementation. My goal isn't to offer medical or professional advice; it is to show you how to work with informed vibration through the chakras to gain optimal benefit from whatever plan you adopt. More detailed information and techniques are in *Advanced Chakra Healing*.

Foods and pH balance: The pH measurement indicates, on a scale of 0 to 14, the balance between acidity and alkalinity in your body. It can be measured using body fluids. Most holistic practitioners I know believe that urine samples reflect physical issues and saliva samples show the presence of emotional issues.

A reading lower than 7.0 reflects more acidity; a reading higher than this number indicates more alkalinity. Many nutritionists and holistic practitioners suggest 7.4 or so as an ideal level, as it is easier for the body to oxygenate when in a slightly alkaline condition. When working the elemental pathway, I recommend you work with a professional to test your pH balance frequently. Use your urine to monitor diet and supplements and your saliva to note mental and emotional strongholds.

Years ago a man named Otto Warburg won a Nobel Prize for showing that cancer thrives in anaerobic or acidic conditions. Research by Keith Brewer, Ph.D., and H. E. Satori has shown that raising the pH, or oxygen content, range of a cell to 8.0 creates a deadly environment for cancer. Common sense, anecdotal evidence, and research are showing the importance of following an acid-free diet when battling cancer.

This diet basically involves eliminating all of the white foods. Take away milk, yeast, all white flours, and sugar, and you've made a good start. Now remove most fruits, white potatoes and rice, corn, coffee, soda pop, alcohol, fruit juices, cheese, junk food, processed soy products, processed meats, high-salt foods, mushrooms, pork, store-bought sauces, hydrogenated or trans fats, saturated fats, and foods with aspartame, hormones, and chemical preservatives, and you're almost there.

What are you supposed to eat? Lots of vegetables, small amounts of proteins to include nonpork flesh, such as beef, chicken, fish, and other seafood, nuts (except for peanuts), healthy oils, legumes, whole grains, and various berries.

It's very difficult to eat "perfectly." That's why it can be so beneficial to work energetically as well as behaviorally. Nutrients bond with energies. The sugar and white flour in cookies may cause temporary physical harm, but if you were constantly shamed when eating cookies as a child, they become charged with the energy of shame. Every time you eat a cookie, you're reinvesting yourself in shame. Or fear, anger, the belief that you are bad—whatever. At the end of the food section, I'll provide an easy-to-use exercise for breaking the bonds between nutrients and harmful energies.

From a pathway perspective, everything said about acidity so far suggests that cancer is largely a negative or electrical condition. Cancer almost always involves a negative component, at least secondarily. What might begin as a positive and alkaline condition over time erodes the rest of your system and creates an acidic environment. However, your originating cancer may be positive, even if the urine doesn't show it. For this indication, you can read the chakra spins as well as your saliva pH to gain a full picture.

The emotional and mental energies attached to your nutrition are reflected in the saliva pH measurement. This measurement will show the presence of emotional versus mental strongholds. An acidic balance in the saliva reflects negative and electrical charges and the corresponding issues of repressed or absorbed feelings and psychic or physical toxins. An alkaline measurement reveals positive and magnetic charges and related spiritual issues. Spiritual issues are more likely to forge as mental strongholds, and power issues as emotional strongholds, though this isn't a hard and fast rule. When I eat chocolate, for instance, my saliva becomes alkaline for at least twenty-four hours, though my urine turns acidic during that entire time. Chocolate carries a spiritual issue for me, although it also sets off a negative spin in my lower chakras.

I'm emphasizing these points because it's important to work all sides of an issue in elemental pathway healing. Don't just "do a diet." Get rid of the charges that make certain foods unhealthy. Better yet, address the exact issues that are creating an alkaline or acidic environment in your primary chakra site, and you stimulate an immediate impact on the cancer.

Metabolic disruptors and assistants: A metabolic disruptor is any substance or nutrient that stops or derails the normal functions of your cells or organs. A metabolic assistant creates or supports the healthy functions of the same. All metabolic food agents fit into one of these four categories: fats, sugars, proteins, and liquids. Other categories include vitamins, minerals, enzymes, and other bodily elements. Most holistic practitioners would say that sugar is a metabolic disruptor and that zinc or some other mineral is a metabolic assistant. In pathway healing, the energy charging a substance is just as important as the actual substance, if not more so. Any nutrient, mineral, vitamin, or substance — even water — could be charged with an energy that harms you. The list of possibilities includes the following:

- Negative spins that make the substance decrease rather than increase power or energy (meaning you'll lose energy with these substances). These nutrients tend to become lodged or stuck in the body and eventually attract "positive" energies such as bacteria or yeast.
- Positive spins that cause substances to reject love or spiritual energies. These nutrients spin out of the body, and you'll experience deficits in regard to these nutrients or properties.
- Absence of spins where there should be spins. A strong misperception can attach to a nutrient and cancel out its healthy properties. Over time, enough stuck "neutered" energies make your chakras stop moving.
- Interference, such as an entity, consciousness, or energetic contract.

Refer to the exercises at the end of this food section to break harmful nutritional bonds and support your nutrients energetically.

Primary chakra sites and related foods: In general, you can boost the healing power of your healthy tissue governed by the primary chakra for the cancer by feeding it with foods that vibrate at its rate. It's important to first charge these foods with helpful information, if you want them to be healing foods. To choose the right foods for you, see *Advanced Chakra Healing*.

Supplements: It is best to consult a professional for a customized assessment of supplements. Your needs change as your cancer changes, so keep your protocol up to date and remember to charge your supplements with helpful information. Supplements that you may want to ask a holistic practitioner about include pancreatic enzyme supplements, emulsified vitamin A, vitamin C complex, vitamin B complex, vitamin P (bioflavonoid), CoQ^{10} essential fats (omega-3 and -6), alpha-lipoic acid, prostaglandins, Essiac, apricot seeds or kernels (controversial and can be poisonous), selenium, maritime pine bark, green and black teas, magnesium oxide, liquid cesium chloride, calcium and magnesium, and amino acids. Your practitioner might recommend milk thistle for liver detoxification, pure cranberry juice for kidney support, shiitake mushrooms for immune-system boosting, wild oregano for yeast detoxification, grape seed extract for viral cleansing, leucozepin compound (found in dong quai and Chinese licorice) to alleviate the effects of chemotherapy and radiotherapy, and several other water-soluble minerals. Specific anti-inflammatory supplements include a combination of the following: pancreatic enzymes, bromelain, vitamin C, papain, quercetin, essential fatty acids, and methylsulfonylmethane (MSM). Also consider the use of homeopathic medicine, Bach Flower Remedies, and other vibrational medicines, if specifically customized to your condition.

Exercises for Food Energy Work

Here are two exercises to connect informed vibration to food for healing.

The "unbonding" exercise: This exercise will free nutrients and inorganic and organic compounds from harmful programs, interference, and bad charges. You can use it for all food properties, liquids, additives, elements, and metabolic disruptors.

1. Center in the sense, feeling, or awareness that results from ingesting a problem food. You may or may not know exactly

what element or compound is causing the problem. It doesn't matter. Acknowledge that something is disturbing your digestive health.

2. Ask to see, hear, or sense which chakra is most affected by this element or compound, then bring your attention to this chakra. If you have a primary cancer site, you could assume this site is the central one.
3. Ask to perceive the element or compound causing difficulties. Now immediately ask to perceive the energy that is bonded to this property and enforcing bodily reactions.
4. Request information about this harmful bond. What do you need to understand? What caused its inception? How is this bond affecting you? Is it primarily related to a belief, feeling, spin, or interference? Now ask what you need to do or to understand to fully and permanently release this harmful bond.
5. Release the bond.
6. Ask what energies you need to activate from deep inside or receive from outside of you to "fill in the gap," to cleanse the bodily area of built-up negative effects, to create a positive relationship with this property, and to strengthen or reinforce the helpful energies of this or any other physical elements or compounds.
7. Check for spin. Are there any changes you now need to transfer into the primary chakra site? Coordinate spin and energies between the property and the chakra, and then close.

Exercise for fortification: You can select any food, supplement, herb, homeopathic remedy, liquid, or product and boost its helpful qualities. You can do the same for medicines, chemotherapy drugs, and radiation. Here is an exercise for fortifying a substance in your body. Basically, this is a way to create a metabolic assistant.

1. Hold the thought, tone, sense, or picture of the selected property in your mind. Ask which chakra vibrates closest to this property's frequency. Bring your consciousness into that chakra.
2. Ask to perceive the energy that will increase the positive and helpful effects of this property in your body in light of a chosen goal. State your goal. Now image, sense, or hear a symbol, color, light, element, number, tone, spin, or any other marker that you will now attach to this property.
3. At what intensity, speed, and spin should this property vibrate to accomplish your goal? If it is supporting a toxic element or compound, ask for an "energy container" so that element will accomplish only the established goal. For example, you may surround the energy of a drug or chemical with an elemental stone wall, so the treatment eliminates only cancer and not healthy cells.
4. Ask the Divine to bless this process and alert you when it's done.

The Role of the Elements The entire physical universe breaks down to ten major elements: water, earth, air, fire, metal, wood, stone, ether, light, and star. Imbalances of any of these elements can create the vibrational disturbances that cause or support cancer; conversely, using or balancing these elements can correct cancerous conditions. Here are the basic properties of the ten elements:

- *Fire:* Eliminates, purges, and burns away. Use fire to purify the blood, lymph system, and infected body areas. Do *not* use on cancer cells; this will backfire and fuel the cancer cells, especially if repressed anger is a component of the cancer.
- *Air:* Transmits ideas and ideals. Use it to "blow away" bad beliefs or initiate helpful ones.
- *Water:* Transmits psychic and feeling energies, soothes and heals, washes and cleanses. Use to cleanse your lymph system or intestines of toxins, both psychic and physical; to

purify the body from chemotherapy and radiation; and to soothe tissue after surgery. Consider programming your drinking water, as explained in the preceding food section.

- *Earth:* Builds, solidifies, and protects; will sustain cell walls and healthy DNA. Imagine yourself filling in mutated DNA with earth energies combined with amino acids. Ask for spiritual genetics to program the earth energies for informed vibration. Use earth energies after surgery to rebuild tissue.
- *Metal:* Protects, defends, and deflects. Use it in the auric field to deflect harmful energies. Establish a metal energetic fort around tumors to keep the cancer from spreading. Purge it from your system if you have heavy metal toxicity; brain and liver cancers often involve a harmful overabundance of metal.
- *Wood:* Adds buoyancy, adaptability, and a positive nature. Insert it in areas of depressed or counterclockwise spin to help set spin clockwise. If depressed emotionally, add it to the mind. Use it to integrate new tissue or ideas into the body, such as after grafts or transplants.
- *Stone:* Strengthens, holds, and toughens. It can be used as a wall around a tumor to keep the body from nourishing the tumor site. Use stone in the tenth chakra to keep the soul grounded in the body. Insert it into the bone tissue for bone cancer. Stone will hold other elements in place; if you need to keep new beliefs anchored so they can root, build a stone retaining wall to do so.
- *Ether:* Holds spiritual truths; can be used to infuse any system, energy body, mind, or soul with such spiritual truths. Use it to bring spiritual truths from the divine pathway into the physical body. These ideas are especially important for spiritually based cancers — for example, those based on beliefs like "It is godly to suffer" or "It's better for me to have cancer than for someone else in my family to have cancer."

- *Light:* Can be directed, spun, fashioned, summoned, or eliminated to produce almost any desired effect. Light is electromagnetic radiations of various wavelengths. Dark light is composed mainly of electrons that carry intelligence about power; "light" light is fashioned chiefly from protons that hold intelligence about love. Bring balance to any off spin with the correct light.
- *Star:* Uses spiritual truths to form and purify physical matter. Burn a spiritual truth into your tissue to reprogram strongholds, change a power field, or alter DNA. Star will also force the release of a misperception or harmful pattern in the body.

Regarding cancer, consider the following use of elements:

- Adding an element to cover deficits
- Adding an element to fill in mutated genes or cell wall weaknesses
- Eliminating elements that feed the cancer itself
- Eliminating elements that perpetuate yeast, viruses, or bacteria

See this chapter's section on "Helpers on the Elemental Pathway" for suggestions on working with elemental beings.

Working with Strongholds The basis of most elemental pathway healing involves breaking strongholds. You might really want to change a pattern but find yourself unable to do so because the energy of the stronghold fixes you in place. Here are initial ways to free your feelings and beliefs. If these don't work, move to the next sections of this chapter and assess for interference and time and space issues. You can also work directly with energy techniques or consider moving to the power pathway, where more intense energies might be holding you stuck.

Freeing Your Feelings Most negatively based cancers involve repressed feelings. You can energetically determine the presence and placement of harmful feelings by looking for counter-clockwise spins, squared-off symbols, dark or bluish energies, and heavy-feeling areas in the body, energy organs, or auric field.

As well, the second chakra records feelings for the entire system. Examine the back side of the second chakra, looking for discolorations, off marks, off tones, or other indications of stored energies. Dark energy lines, which are actually internal cords, will track to the entry or storage site of these feelings. Also assess the inner wheel of the second chakra. If it is overtly spinning in reverse, either this or another chakra is holding repressed feelings. These feelings might have originated with you, others, or both.

Before you can work with your own feelings, get rid of others' energies using the releasing exercises under "Freeing Yourself from Others' Energies and Interference" in the chapter 5 insert. Center in your primary cancer chakra, then use the "Healing Feelings" exercise in the insert to release the feeling, figure out its message, and undo the stronghold.

Healing Your Beliefs Bad beliefs come from the past. You may have personally determined them or simply absorbed them from others. Harmful beliefs are primarily stored in the electrons — which initiate structure — and therefore these beliefs affect your sense of power. In cases involving negative cancers, your life is designed around these harmful beliefs. In cases of positive cancers, the programming in the protons determines your ability to give and receive love. If your beliefs disregard the importance of love, your own body won't "love itself" enough to eliminate cancer. Neutron-based cancers involve a single belief, which establishes a universal pattern that affects all of your life. Change the belief creating the cancer and you can change your entire life.

Bad beliefs can eventually erode healthy physical and energetic systems. Inserting healthy and loving beliefs into our chakras, bodies, minds, and cells can enable positive restructuring and genetic reprogramming.

Here is a simple exercise to alter a belief-based pattern. Conduct it after you have determined whether or not you are currently taking on beliefs from others, as discussed in the chapter 5 insert.

1. Center in the chakra holding the originating belief or belief stronghold. If you have cancer, reference the chakra that is your primary chakra site. Otherwise, you can check for the affected chakra via your third or seventh chakra. Through the back side of the third, you can track energy lines to the conflicted chakra. Through the seventh chakra's pineal gland, you can observe dark, light, or red energies in all chakras that show strongholds. Dark indicates an electron basis; light, a proton basis; and red, a neutron basis. As well, check for spin and color in various chakras. Dark and reverse spins reveal electrons and probably emotional strongholds; light and clockwise spins indicate protons and, typically, mental strongholds; red and stuck spins mean neutrons and a single, foundational misperception.
2. Use the insert table of power levels and fields in *Advanced Chakra Healing* to get a sense of which types of beliefs are causing you problems. Refer to the listing of beliefs in the insert (under "Energy Absorption Issues") to further define your harmful beliefs.
3. Ask your intuition or the Divine to clarify the original misperception or set of beliefs causing the stronghold. You will hear, sense, or see an answer. Ask to understand the origin of the belief. At what age did you initiate or accept this belief? In what lifetime? For what reason? What contract is keeping it in place? Are you holding this agreement with another person or energy, or primarily with yourself (as in the case of a codependent contract, which loops inside of yourself but affects all your relationships)? How has this belief or stronghold affected your life? How has it affected the cancer?

4. Ask now what you need to understand or do to release the misperceptions and initiate a helpful belief. Deep inside are the beliefs you are meant to have; these are based on spiritual truths. What needs to happen to allow these to come forth and assume their rightful authority? Ask other questions as you see fit, and follow the advice provided.

Basic Energy Healing: Special Elemental Techniques

Elemental pathway healing involves our basic concepts of working energetically. By reducing your diagnosis to electrical or negative, positive or magnetic, or neutron or neutral, you can tap into the world of informed vibration and use the following concepts for healing: particles and waves, spin, color, shapes, tones, and forces and fields. Included in this section are a few exercises for improving the success of traditional treatments.

Particle and Wave Healing Recall that particles can turn into waves and vice versa. Waves generate a much stronger field than do particles. Use these facts to your advantage in the following ways:

- Cancer cells are particles, though their overwhelming abilities suggest that they are drawing power from waves that are harmful to your body. With intention, chakra-based meditation, or use of vibrational medicines such as homeopathy, cancel out the harmful wave by calling forth a wave from your own spirit. This second wave will harmonize to your body and will naturally be more powerful than any subversive energy.
- Healthy cells are particles. Their energetics, however, can be transformed into a waveform. Use intention to free a healthy cell's energy, so it works like a wave. Intensify this wave and direct it at cancer particles, thus overwhelming them.

- Many negative cancers are linked to viruses, which often link to group consciousness waves. To deal directly with an underlying virus, call forth a spiritual truth available on the divine pathway or through a spiritual point. Turn this truth into a wave to eliminate the virus.
- Many positive cancers connect with yeast, mold, and bacteria. When these grow in the body, they encourage the development of acidity, which then generates negative energies in the body. Yeast, mold, and bacteria exist in the presence of spiritual assumptions that are self-defeating and damaging. Psychically examine these microbes for the consciousness wave that carries the destructive ideas. Bring in a wave of truth to change the ideas.
- For potent healing of neutral cancers, erase the cancer-causing, harmful belief in the center of the cell that carries it. Substitute a wave of truth for this particle that is a lie.

Spin Check the primary cancer site for incorrect spin, then use your intuition to figure out the correct spin. Once you've established correct spin, lock it in with a symbol. You can select an appropriate symbol, number, or tone after conducting the chapter 7 exercise for figuring out your harmonic. And you can always turn to the Divine to select a lock for you, or you can test a symbol psychically and see if it holds.

Once you have altered your primary chakra, check all other chakras and set their spins correctly. Check for rhythm inside each chakra and between all chakras.

You can also alter the spins of your cancer cells. What can you do to disrupt their spins? Sometimes you have only to bring order to their erratic spins, and the body will recognize the cancer cells as mutant and destroy them.

One interesting technique for changing spins is to do so on X-rays or scans instead of on the body. Hold your pendulum over the X-ray or scan to assess for spin. Use intention to change the pattern on your scan, then ask the Divine to transfer the necessary healing energies into your body to permanently create this change. I know a man who had a brain tumor and used toning to conduct this type of healing. He toned on his MRI scan for healing and asked that these correct tones be transmitted into his head. The next time he was checked for cancer, the tumor was gone.

Color As described in the insert, you can work with color diagnostically or for healing. Color healing, however, can get complicated. Here is my advice.

Psychically, a healthy electron state is deep rich ebony. A negatively based cancer will appear as blue, often cobalt in hue, or a brackish dark color. As strange as it sounds, you can ask the Divine to provide you the correct hue of black when working with negative cancers. The correct black will restore a chakra to its accurate color; for instance, before a healing, a cancer-ridden fourth chakra might be an off green. Healthy black will refresh this chakra to a bright green.

Positive cancers usually appear a strange, milky white or an off yellow. Gold is the sign of healthy protons and a good color to work with for positive-based cancers.

Neutral cancers will reflect red tones rather than the pink seen in a healthy neutron. Shades of pink or rose are best applied in neutral cancers.

Shape Use the lists of shapes in the insert to evaluate the shapes in your primary chakra sites. If you've removed an unhealthy one during your work, be sure to replace it with a new shape. In general, circular shapes establish healthy relationships, square shapes offer protection, pyramid shapes will restore the ability to manifest, and spirals will create release or attraction. A cross with a circle is always a good shape for locking in a beneficial change.

Numbers can also be useful. Someone who is lonely will have a numeral 1 in their chakra centers. By simply substituting the numeral 2,you enable the person to attract partnership.

Tones If you are an auditory psychic, toning can be of great benefit. Figure out your personal spiritual harmonic, as detailed in chapter 7. Once you know your harmonic, you'll intuitively know which tones are healthy for you and which ones are not.

In general, lower-frequency tones can help break up negative cancers, higher-frequency tones can pierce positive cancers, and middle-range tones can help reprogram neutral cancers. For potent toning, vibrate tones in octaves. For instance, play a low and a high C to work with a negative cancer. This creates a harmonic that distorts the cancer frequency at its lower and higher ends.

Forces and Fields We've considered many energetic variables, yet an entire library could be created out of information about forces and fields. Here are a few suggestions that pertain to cancer.

There are many types of natural forces. A complete list is outlined in *Advanced Chakra Healing: Energy Mapping*. Check and see which is fueling the cancer. A weak nuclear force? Gravity? You can obtain this answer by working psychically in your primary chakra site. Now ask your spiritual guides or the Divine to tell you how to combat the relationship between the cancer and the force. Which alternative force might disrupt the cancer's bonding? Which will free you of cancer? Consider supplementing helpful natural forces with spiritual energetic forces from the power pathway (see chapter 7).

Here are a few ways to use personal fields and external fields for your cancer battle.

Personal Fields The magnetic field you generate to heal from cancer must be high powered, as the magnetic field provides the basis for strength and intensity for your entire energy system and therefore your physical body. To increase the power of your magnetic field, eliminate all energies draining your electrical energies, such as repressed feelings and psychic or physical toxins. Then, centering in your heart, ask the Divine to join its will with your willpower; decide that you will now generate your magnetic field at 100 percent capacity. The Divine will automatically boost you to 100 percent, but internal issues and fears can prevent your system from sustaining this increase, which is why it is best to first address electrical issues.

Auric Fields With the auric fields, for the most part you energetically work as you would with the chakras. Check for energetic contracts, possession or recession, absorption of other energies, and all other matters. Use regression, projecting, or futuring to further define the origination issues and vibrational means to heal. For cancer, attend to the following particular issues:

Holes: Auric holes allow in energies that are psychically or physically carcinogenic. If there is a hole in the field related to your primary cancer site, it is probably bleeding you of basic life energy and filling you with carcinogens. When closing holes, make sure you first release any stored negative energies from the body.

Weak spots: Weakened, thin, light-colored, or soft auric areas mirror the "mushy" nature of the precancerous cells. Before a cell completely mutates, the vital force within it begins to wane. Strengthen these weak spots with tonal or color therapy and lock the changes in symbolically.

Discoloration: You might spot colors that don't fit in this field, are muddied, or are otherwise disturbed. These off hues mirror the conditions causing problems in the chakras. Some discolorations reflect the mutations on the cancer genes; if this is the case, access the spiritual genetics on the power pathway, as described in chapter 7. Then transfer these spiritual energies into your physical genes before fully correcting your auric field.

Symbology issues: Like the chakras, the auric bands can show symbols. Look carefully to observe whether any of these representations are linked or corded to the cancerous mass in the body. If so, these symbols reinforce the cancerous condition and might even have been the original primary site, as in cases in which a curse penetrated the field. Change the symbol and establish a new one in the pertinent chakra and auric field.

Off tones: The aurally gifted can hear the tones of the various auric fields and perceive variations. An aberrant tone can be changed by listening to correct music, chanting, or humming. You can even picture the correct note and insert it into the field.

Interference: With few exceptions, interference that's obvious within a chakra will be visible within an auric field. You can work in either place to challenge and change this interference.

External Fields Ley lines are fields of electromagnetic energies in the earth. They are part of the family of Vivaxis energies — energetic lines and networks that connect all living things with electromagnetic energies found in and above the earth. Your family lineage might be corded to a ley line running on unhealthy soil or over radioactive material, which can generate cancer in your body. For negative cancers, check to see if you are hooked into a highly electrical ley line or any other electrical field, such as those from a planet or a star. For positive cancers, evaluate for highly magnetic ley lines or other Vivaxis connections. Regarding neutral cancers, look to see if you need to be connected to a certain type of electromagnetic line to activate your healing abilities.

Know too that you can deliberately link into the variety of Vivaxis lines for healing purposes. If you have a negative cancer, how about grounding into a source of magnetic frequencies, such as those carried in valleys, dales, and streams? If you have a positive cancer, consider flooding your body with negative fields, such as those obtained on mountaintops and high points on the earth.

Working in the Power Field Playing with the power field is a powerful way to pop off of strongholds. *Power fields* are a progressive order of energetic fields that stair-step you through the human development process into owning your divinity. A complete outline of power levels and power fields is available in *Advanced Chakra Healing*. Playing with the power field is a powerful way to pop off of strongholds.

The Inner Child Comes Out to Play I am a firm believer in working through inner-child issues to heal from cancer. Your inner children are aspects of yourself that have been traumatized. These aspects of the self remain stuck in time and energetically continue to experience the initial trauma until they are freed and healed.

Energetically, the presence of a trapped inner child produces the same stress on the body as a deep splinter. The inner child and its feelings, beliefs, and corded energies will be interpreted as a foreign object by the body, which will either attack it and create inflammation or change the DNA so it matches the energies being expressed in or around the hidden child. As psychologically challenging as it may be to admit, *cancer often occurs because the body mirrors the energies trapping the hidden inner child or alters the DNA to match those of this hidden self.*

If you have cancer, you *must* free your internal inner child.

Inner-child work involves gaining the trust of the secreted self and finding out his or her story. You must then rescue this child, which ultimately frees the stuck energy and allows the chakra to reestablish health. An inner child is frequently involved in an emotional stronghold and sometimes in a mental stronghold.

Many healers orient healing by looking for soul issues, karmic patterns carried over from past lives. Inner children mirror soul issues, which is part of the reason working the inner-child realm is so powerful. Past-life trauma is sometimes the reason that a this-life child draws an experience to itself. (This does *not* mean that you are responsible for abuse you suffered! Abusers are always responsible for their own actions.) A soul trauma affects the energy system, leaving holes and strongholds that keep you from knowing how to create safety. When you heal an inner child, you heal the soul and pave the way for attracting powerful spiritual energies that magnify healing.

Here are the basic steps involved in reaching and helping an inner child:

1. In the case of cancer, begin work in the primary site. Check for indications of an inner child, as noted above.
2. Ask to communicate with this child. Have it show you what occurred to cause the fear. Upon receiving the story, ask the inner child how its presence has been affecting your life.
3. To help the child self, ask it what is needed. Usually, the need is to be rescued from the threat, which from the child's perspective is still occurring. Call upon the Divine, guardian angels, or your own future or higher self to help address the threat.
4. Upon removing the child from the scene of the trauma, ask the Divine where this child needs to be kept to keep it safe until "grown up." Cleanse the trauma site energetically or have a spiritual guide do it.
5. Check for cords, especially connected to the abuser. Also evaluate for codependent cords or life-energy cords to a past life. Use the cord exercise in the insert to deal with these.
6. Establish the correct spin patterns in the chakra before closing.

Dealing with Interference As explained in the insert, interference is any form of energy or entity that keeps you from living in your own truth. Energetically, it establishes a vibration or set of vibrations that inhibit your own harmonic. When working on the elemental pathway, you should check the following places or sites for energetic contracts, entities, group consciousness, hauntings, or other interference, including areas in which you absorb others' energies:

- Chakras, auric fields, and other energy bodies
- Organs affected by cancer
- Cells and growths that are cancerous
- Lymph system near primary or secondary cancer sites
- Foods, supplements, or liquids commonly consumed
- Morphogenetic field
- Inside of the energy egg or between the layers of the energy egg — interference between the first and second layer can prevent realization of your dreams for healing; between the second and third layer can deflect healing spiritual energies
- Into any part or aspect of the self

If interference is present, use the exercises listed in the insert section "Freeing Yourself from Others' Energies and Interference" to clear it.

Kundalini: The Serpent Rising In cases of cancer, kundalini on the elemental pathway is nearly always depressed. Kundalini expresses itself as a serpent that rises through the body. It appears red, as it is composed of basic life energy. Cancer actually leaches the basic life energy of the tissues in the primary cancer site. The body recognizes only that the basic life energy is still present, not noting that aberrant cells are misusing it. The body therefore fails to summon additional basic life energy. The kundalini, a product of the first chakra in men and second chakra in women, remains at a low ebb. The types of strongholds underlying cancer can also stifle the serpent kundalini.

To gain the basic life energy needed to fight cancer, you must raise the kundalini. Follow the exercises in *Advanced Chakra Healing* for working your kundalini.

Time and Space Travels Sometimes cancer is related to occurrences on other dimensions or realms. An aspect of the self might be caught in another spacetime. It might be corded to an entity or energy that dwells elsewhere. It might have originally incurred damage somewhere else or at some other time, and it needs to return to this spacetime to release the trauma or reclaim a lost energy. Sometimes several parts of us exist simultaneously, and we need to bring an interdimensional aspect into the here and now to recover from cancer. Or we might simply need the advice or healing energies from a being from elsewhere!

Connecting to another spacetime is no more difficult than thinking about another room in your house. Use processes described in the insert, such as the Projection Exercise or the Regression Exercise, to visit another spacetime. You can also use the insert's "Five Steps for Safe Psychic Use"; after opening, simply ask to experience the spacetime needed to understand. It's often easiest to conduct this connection through the eighth chakra or by using an imagination mirror on the imagination pathway (see chapter 8). In cases involving cancer, remain centered in the primary cancer chakra and ask to intuitively perceive the important information while within this area. Conduct your healing as indicated. There are various types of places and spaces. A complete description of these is available in *Advanced Chakra Healing: Energy Mapping*.

Dimensions There are thirteen main dimensions. Basically, the easiest way to access any of them is through the eighth chakra or through the chakra that corresponds numerically. For instance, you get to the first dimension through the first chakra. The higher dimensions enable you to integrate other pathways into elemental pathway work. To get into a dimension, center yourself in the middle of the selected chakra and ask the Divine to link you. First refer to the information in *Advanced Chakra Healing* that describes each dimension and ways to work within them, then ask to see or sense the energies supporting the cancer.

Planes of Light When the body dies, the soul passes through twelve planes into a final thirteenth to merge back into spirit. You can access the healing energies of any of these planes and transfer them into your body at will. Read about the planes in *Advanced Chakra Healing*, then use "Five Steps for Safe Psychic Use" to do this.

Zones of Life and Death There are several zones that assist the soul in its alchemical processes between life, death, and the space in between lives. To access one of these zones, use the eighth chakra or center yourself in the primary cancer chakra and ask the Divine to connect you with any one of these zones. You can also use journeying techniques such as regression to recall your progression through any of these zones.

- *The White Zone:* The space without time, in which the soul determines upcoming life goals, lessons, and events. Go here to figure out various reasons you might have pre-arranged for cancer before this lifetime, and whether you can and should change the plan.
- *The Gray Zone:* The place where space and time meet while the soul is exiting the White Zone and beginning its entry orbit into an awaiting body. Here you potentially gather interference that can steal your basic life energy. Check here for cords and eliminate them.
- *The Red Zone:* The place where space and time meet while the soul is still lingering in the body, but just about to exit into the Black Zone. You still have some of your basic life energy in this state. If you are exhausted and believe that you could better battle cancer if you had more energy, return here to reclaim what you are missing.

- *The Black Zone:* The space without time just after death in which the soul pauses before deciding which way to go through the Planes of Light. Sometimes part of the soul gets stuck here, and you must reclaim it to fill in missing holes in your energy system. Other times it creates cords or attachments, which could be underlying the conditions of a malignancy. Release all attachments that you find.

Helpers on the Elemental Pathway

On the elemental pathway, you can call on helpers from all levels of reality. Here are a partial list and the best methods for accessing each category for healing cancer. Detailed descriptions of these sources are provided in *Advanced Chakra Healing*.

The Natural World Call upon the beings of the natural world to support your healing process.

- *Ancestors:* Can be summoned to alter inherited DNA coding
- *Power animals and totems:* Can provide information and healing energies
- *Plant spirits:* Can infuse your body with their own energies
- *Nature beings:* Can cleanse your environment — this is especially useful with cancers caused by environmental poisons, but everyone benefits from cleared space
- *Beings of earth, the stars, and planets:* Can support your healthy cells and reinforce your immune system

Elemental Beings Elemental beings can help balance your body and pH, supply missing elements and nutrients, and detoxify as well.

- *Water beings:* Can purge your system of poisons
- *Fire beings:* Can burn up yeast, mold, fungus, and sometimes

less intense feelings such as sadness (differentiated from sorrow) and frustration (differentiated from rage or anger); used strategically, fire beings can eliminate toxins and waste products

- *Metal beings:* Can provide protection — for instance, by propping them like walls around healthy tissue when you are undergoing chemotherapy
- *Stone beings:* Can offer fortification and strength; use them to keep your soul in your body during surgery or when under intense stress; they are also useful in bone cancers, as they can fill in the areas consumed by cancer
- *Wood beings:* Can clarify an area; use them to clear the "deadwood" out of an infested or cancerous body part
- *Earth beings:* Can fill in the organic tissues of your body — for instance, to help your body repair after surgery
- *Air beings:* Carry information and can alter programming wherever they are placed; you can transform cancer cells by inserting air beings with healthy codes directly into the malignant cells
- *Light beings:* Summon a light being to alter the cancerous DNA coding or to enable healthy cells to continue to divide in correct ways
- *Ether beings:* Can provide diagnostic information or summon spiritual energies from beyond the energy egg for your well-being
- *Star beings:* Can cleanse and reeducate cells or tissues simultaneously, which means they can both kill cancer cells and reprogram healthy cells that could mutate

Human Sources These helpers include people living and dead. Here are ways to tap into their extraordinary assistance.

- Ask the Divine to source you into the spirit of a well-known healer to access his or her knowledge.

- Ask the Divine to source you into someone who has been healed of the type of cancer you have. Ask that the energy that healed him or her be transmitted to you through divine love.
- Ask for a guide from the past or the future who knows how to heal cancer.
- Remember the living! Your friends, family, and professional contacts are all members of your support system. Let them help you.

Aspects of the Self There are many ways to access your own current, past, or potential knowledge.

- *The God self:* The self you would have been if raised with the Divine as your parents. Ask the God self to transmit healing and knowledge from this already-healthy self.
- *The primal self:* The part of you devoted solely to self-preservation. For example, allow your primal self to heal your DNA.
- *The innocent child:* The self who was never harmed by life experiences, those incurred in this or any other lifetime. He or she can use transmission to attend to the wounded inner children and return them to wholeness.
- *The future self:* The self who has already healed from cancer. Allow him or her to attend to you and show you which healing paths result(ed) in full recovery.
- *The master self:* Selves that have specific gifts and abilities. Determine your need and ask that a master self step forward to assist.
- *The higher self:* The self that understands fully the reasons for the cancer but holds no judgment. This self uses the power of compassion to transmit healing energies.

In addition to these selves, the High Heart can heal the deep emotional and relationship wounds and therefore emotional strongholds of the Low Heart. The High Mind can erase the erroneous assumptions forging mental strongholds in the Low Mind.

Finally, you can invite your own spirit to access the spiritual energies that will heal you. You are your spirit and can therefore heal yourself!

Spiritual Sources Spiritual sources serve the Divine. It is best to ask the Divine to assign you the guides that can best help you and to ask for the same to assist your care providers. These sources might be living or deceased. They include masters, avatars, saints, gurus, sorcerers (of white magic), shamans, healers, and allies, as well as the last two types of forms. As described initially in chapter 2, there is a group of beings naturally gifted in transferring energy from one state to another. There are also beings who learn this skill in relation to a specific craft. In the Divine, both types of forms are in attendance. And of course, invite the angels. Angels may or may not be invested with the power to "cure your cancer," but they can deliver messages; provide knowledge, direction, comfort, and inspiration; and guide you toward other helpful sources.

chapter seven

Energy Mapping on the Power Pathway

But there is something strange about all these blondes.
Very few of them are genuine.

—Joanna Pitman, *On Blondes*[1]

Travel the power pathway under these conditions:

- You have a precancerous condition, or know which body sites or chakras are primary to the cancer
- You can sense, see, or verbally interpret the presence of unseen forces
- You are interested in supernatural or controlling forces and energies
- You believe that these can be commanded for gain
- You often work with chakra five, eight, or eleven

The Power Pathway: Brawn over Brain

It's a known fact that very few adult women with blonde hair are actually blonde at the roots. Some substance has altered the appearance of the hair, seemingly by magic! Women know that they must continually reapply this "magic potion" to maintain the effect. What if you could defy this law of reapplication? What if you could apply the coloring agent only once and it would stay?

On the power pathway, this is entirely possible.

The power pathway is the access vehicle for spiritual energies and forces that lock physical reality in place. You could decide to stick a degenerative spiritual force on a chakra, for instance, and this force would suck energy out of that chakra forevermore. You could decide to stick this same force on a tumor and vacuum the cancer right out of it. No one judges what you do with the forces available through this pathway. Once you put a power pathway force in place, however, it will operate until you change it again.

Once you know about the powers accessible on this pathway, you can check for forces in place and change them at will. You don't have to identify the deeper meaning of every problem or issue. On this pathway, brawn is more important than brain; muscle meets the mind. You do have to know what to look for, however, and to claim your capability of commanding for change.

Cancer and the Power Pathway

Cancer is a tricky disease in the physical realm, and it is no different on the power pathway. The key to working the power pathway for supportive cancer healing is to search until you find the exact forces that are allowing the cancer to reign and keeping healthy cells deranged.

Working the *spiritual energetic forces* — the summative phrase to describe the various energies available on the power pathway —

lends you superhuman qualities. Once you figure out exactly which forces need to be activated and which forces need to be deactivated, you can take the vim out of cancer and renew the vigor in your healthy cells. It's like being an electrician. If you plug in a lamp and turn on the switch, you have light. Unplug from the socket or turn off the switch, the lamp turns off. So it is with cancer. What forces are supporting the energies that are feeding your cancer and turning its light on? Switch off these forces and your body's ability to nourish the cancer dies. It's helpful to simultaneously initiate the bodily energies that nurture your healthy cells and your immune system. This way your natural body functions can do their job and wipe out the cancer.

There are two basic steps to working with the power pathway for intense healing:

1. Identify which spiritual energetic forces need to be turned off and unplugged.
2. Identify which forces need to be plugged in and turned on.

Tools and Healing on the Power Pathway

These are the energies and principles available for healing cancer on this pathway:

- Energies on the Power Pathway
- The Main Principle of Command: Resonance
- Special Power Pathway Techniques
- Helpers on the Power Pathway

Energies on the Power Pathway

I want to introduce you to the energy bodies and spiritual energetic forces of the power pathway that I think will be most useful in your efforts against cancer.

The primary power pathway energy bodies are the seals, which are connected with your chakras. There are many other power pathway energy bodies (described in detail in *Advanced Chakra Healing: Energy Healing*), but I'm going to concentrate on the seals, as these are the most effective tools regarding cancer.

The seals look like lenses that attach to each chakra on the front side and the backside. Why are the seals shaped like lenses? If you work a lens just right, you can focus energy through its center point and direct it at will. That's exactly what we want to do with a seal. We want to channel power pathway energies through the center of each lens for our own well-being.

When we're born, the convex sides of each lens usually face outward. In this position, we have little to no control over the energies that each lens is attracting or disseminating. Hence our seals are either ineffective in managing the supernatural energies available on the power, or are using energies that reinforce our innate or learned programming (which includes all our harmful programs). At some point, we (hopefully) reach the emotional and spiritual maturation necessary to use the seals more consciously and conscientiously. At this point, we might knowingly or unknowingly "set a seal," which involves flipping the lenses connected to a chakra so the convex side faces the chakra center point. We can set one or more seal at a time, or all at once. Once set, the concave bowl is able to receive the spiritual energies of the universe and the convex side focuses powers for personal use.

The seals transmit high-intensity energies and activate only when you are able to command their powers. Through the seals, you can generate the potency needed to reinforce the energies that support healthy cellular functions and eliminate the forces holding the cancer in place.

On the power pathway, you can use the chakras as you do on the elemental pathway, or you can supplement this work with the seals. Using the seals adds speed and thrust to your work. You can also read the center of a seal to examine it for spiritual energetic forces.

Here are descriptions of each seal and its primary relationship to cancer.

Seal One: Brings spiritual matter into the physical body. This can nourish areas weak from cancer or chemotherapy with new energies or create healthy cells that can battle the cancer.

Seal Two: Connects with feelings in forces. All power pathway forces have feeling energies in them. This seal naturally attracts forces that can help you quickly release the feelings underlying cancer or give you the emotional boost you need to maintain commitment to healing. Can fast-track the release of others' feelings supporting the cancer.

Seal Three: Works with consciousness waves instead of only thoughts. Consciousness waves are strong bands of thoughts that can implement immediate change in beliefs and ideas. They can "change your mind" as easily as they can convert the data on a malignant DNA cell to conform to healthy standards.

Seal Four: Focuses divine love. Can call on various spiritual energetic forces — like virtues and overall energy of divine love — to bring relationships into balance. Cancer is "out of relationship" with the rest of the body; this seal supports the cancer cells in conforming to the body or supports the rest of the body in eliminating these abnormal cells.

Seal Five: Boosts verbal vibrations for immediate healing. Bring the energies from spiritual guides directly into the body for healing purposes and focuses tones or messages to reprogram the DNA or the surrounding cells.

Seal Six: Activates visual information so it forms a template right in the body. You can hold an image of your desired healing and, through the seal, attach a force that sends this image into form so the body has no choice but to conform. Enables you to command change in the body as soon as you perceive a solution.

Seal Seven: Imprints consciousness and spiritual waves directly into the body. By "forcing" a new consciousness, you can convert the body to a more desirable state. By initiating spiritual energies into the body, you form it to its destined state, which is ideally healthy. Allows for full transmission of consciousness from your spiritual guides, so you can, for instance, accept a healing master's standard of health.

Seal Eight: Aligns here and now with potential from other planes and worlds. One method is to first select the image of a healed self from another dimension, then focus power pathway forces to align the physical body with this potential. Another technique is to summon energies or healers from other planes and assist them with the spiritual energetic forces needed to heal you from cancer. You can potentially bring the energy of a cancer-curing drug back in time from the future and hook it into your body right now! A different method involves hooking power pathway forces up to the elemental pathway nutrients (such as herbs or supplements) used to battle the cancer. This "oomph" greatly increases the effectiveness of your healing.

Seal Nine: Activates principles directly into the body. For example, a soul might undertake cancer because it wants to point out the societal danger of power lines. Is this a higher-order principle, if the one suffers for the all? Through the power pathway, you can stimulate a more advanced principle such as "Everyone deserves to be healthy" and force the body to conform to this principle instead of the other.

Seal Ten: Awakens full consciousness and energetic vibrations of natural-world energies and beings. Read what you can accomplish through the tenth chakra, then think of what could happen if you magnify the effects of your connections by a hundred. Through the tenth seal, you can do just that. You can increase the potency of an herb a hundredfold and apply a power pathway force that is a hundred times faster at wiping out yeast. Likewise, you can detoxify from the effects of chemotherapy. Also, you can raise your "consciousness connection" to animate beings multifold. Let's say you need the energy of a hawk to keep you committed to a cancer-reducing diet. Focusing a power pathway force on "hawk" raises your vibration to hold the goal-setting abilities of "hawk."

Seal Eleven: What might happen if you could instantly vibrate natural or supernatural energies from zero to one hundred in amplitude within moments? That's the potential when focusing commands through the eleventh seal. The challenge is to make sure you are calling forces through *resonance*, using vibration to discern which forces fit with which goals.

Seal Twelve: Interfaces with all layers of the energy egg to draw forces that alleviate our human concerns. The divine energy within us, through the twelfth seal, can call through resonance to all the forces on the power pathway. Commanding rather than begging for help asserts the power of love, and the help appears where we need it.

Two other energy bodies are especially beneficial when addressing cancer. The etheric mirror or Christ body (introduced in chapter 6) contains the programming for our perfect, healthy body. The other helpful energy body directly linked with the power pathway is the *Book of Life*. Similar to the Akashic Records (see chapter 8), this reservoir of knowledge contains everything you've ever done or experienced in the past, present, or potential future but only through the perspective of love. Later in this chapter I offer exercises that use both of these energy bodies for healing cancer.

The Spiritual Energetic Forces on the Power Pathway Spiritual energetic forces consist of multiple energies. Some are quanta-based; others are magnetic, electrical, or electromagnetic. Some are formed of pure consciousness and are aware and alive; others emanate from different planets or worlds. The variety can seem scary and overwhelming. How do you know what these superhuman energies might do to you?

Have no fear. I've included a section that teaches you about resonance — a way to discover which forces will assist rather than hurt — followed by a short section on methods that will help keep you from accidentally creating problems or causing harm when using spiritual energetic forces.

Here is a list of the basic spiritual energetic forces. For a more thorough explanation of each, see *Advanced Chakra Healing: Energy Mapping.*

- *Spiritual forces:* These energies lock into parts of the energy system or the body to either remove or add energy. Degenerative spiritual forces take energy away, whereas generative spiritual forces add energy. These aren't "bad" or "good" energies, merely properties that create an effect. The degenerative force of chaos, for instance, could also break up a tumor so your body can dissolve it. The generative force of regeneration could renew a tired liver, but could also cause cancer cells to multiply uncontrollably.
- *Powers:* Of course there has to be something called "powers" on the power pathway! The powers are named the same as the elements: fire, water, earth, air, wood, metal, stone, ether, light, and star. These powers are elementally based energies that come from the spiritual realms that attach to the spiritual forces. They give a certain spin or quality to the connected force. Take the degenerative spiritual force of chaos; the fire energy can enable it to burn away the toxic waste produced by cancer cells.

- *Virtues:* Virtues are energies holding ideals. They can shape your chakras and beliefs to conform to the concepts they represent. With a virtue, it isn't a matter of good or bad; it's about fit or lack of fit. The virtue of goodness might be connected to a mental stronghold that it's "good to suffer"; therefore, cancer might be the solution for the person searching for a reason to suffer. The same virtue of goodness could attach to the throat chakra and encourage you to eat only foods that are good for you, thus keeping you on a cancer-preventive diet. Virtues plug into the chakra back sides.
- *Rays:* Rays are multidimensional energies that connect one chakra to another to help them attain ideal functioning. The ray of will, for instance, bolsters the best ideas of the first chakra, and it can keep you on target when you decide to heal from cancer.
- *Golden kundalini:* Golden kundalini is a process (described in the insert) for raising the red serpent kundalini to a spiritual level. This process magnifies the healing properties of your body and alerts you to your spiritual abilities.

The Main Principle of Command: Resonance

Commanding is the means of moving energy on the power pathway. To command, you must assume the right to command.

Do you know that each of us is invested with the authority to design our own welfare? This *doesn't* mean that we are singularly responsible for all the bad things that happen to us in life, even getting cancer. We aren't responsible for all the good things, either. We're interdependent, not only with other people but also with all of nature and the greater universe. Just as you get to turn off the television when you're done watching, however, so are you able to turn power pathway forces on or off.

Now, you don't want to turn off the television at the wrong time. What if you've been waiting hours to see a certain program, and you switch it off only moments before it comes on? What if there are other people in the room? Have you ever aborted a child's favorite cartoon right in the middle of the most important episode? It's important to know which power pathway forces to shift in or out and when to turn them on or off. There's a very specific law that will help you know what to command and how: the *Law of Resonance.*

There are two basic meanings to the word *resonance*. One refers to the vibration produced in an object (or person or energy) when subjected to vibration from another source that is at or near its natural frequency. The other refers to the ability of certain chemical compounds to hold the characteristics of two or more electronic structures at the same time.

Here's how we apply these ideas for healing cancer. In relation to the definition of resonance, *we want to work with energies that resonate with our wholeness rather than our brokenness.* Unfortunately, treatments such as chemotherapy seldom resonate with our healthy, harmonic self. On the power pathway, you have the opportunity to call on spiritual energetic forces that bolster your natural harmonic rather than increase dissonance. You could even use spiritual energetic forces to bolster the work of the chemotherapy and help the chemicals resonate better with your harmonic.

To accomplish goals for resonance:

1. If you're verbally adept, psychically listen to the tone of your spiritual harmonic. You will be discovering this tone in the next section of this chapter. Get rid of spiritual energetic forces that don't match; use only those that do.
2. If you're visually gifted, psychically compare a spiritual energetic force with the coloration, hue, symbol, or other pictorial representation of your spiritual harmonic. Use forces that match or bolster your harmonic; purge yourself of ones that do not.

3. If you're kinesthetic — meaning you employ chakras one, two, three, four, seven, nine, ten, and eleven — then sense, feel, smell, taste, or touch your spiritual harmonic in comparison with a spiritual energetic force. This will tell you what matches or doesn't.

In relation to the second idea of resonance, *we want to disrupt the resonance of cancer*. Cancer qualifies as the second type of resonating energies; it can perform two different tasks at the same time and hold two different types of energies at the same time. Whether they know it or not, this is one of the reasons that traditional medical doctors use chemotherapy and radiation. They are attempting to disturb the internal resonance of a cancer cell so it is destroyed or so the body is then able to destroy it.

Cancer, with its dualistic resonance, chokes off healthy cells while keeping itself oxygenated. It kills off its host while keeping itself alive. It convinces the physical body to nourish it while staying hidden from the immune system. Cancer cells are cells that have destroyed their own DNA, yet this is the basis of their own existence. And *cancer cannot survive unless able to continually perform its seemingly opposite tasks in an ongoing fashion.* If the cancer vibrationally shifted to allow healthy cells to oxygenate or to recognize the existence of the cancer, the healthy cells would destroy the cancer.

Do you want to disrupt the resonance of cancer? Attune to spiritual energetic forces that will slice the beast in half! Try the following:

1. If you're verbally gifted, connect with your own spiritual harmonic. Now ask your spiritual guides to attune you to the single frequency within that harmonic, or an overtone or undertone that will disrupt the cancer. You might hear the answer in a word or phrase, such as "F sharp." Go buy music written in the key of F sharp. You might hear a tone. Hum and match it. However you get the message, ask that this tone

be matched with a spiritual energetic force that will increase its potency so the cancer cannot hold its own resonance.

2. If you're visually adept, image your spiritual harmonic. Now ask the Divine or your spiritual guides to formulate one single image that will break the resonance of the cancer in two. Use your guidance to again match this image with the corresponding, resonant spiritual energetic forces and translate these into a picture of the cancer held in your mind's eye.
3. If you are primarily kinesthetic, select your favored way to sense reality. Connect into your sensation or knowing of your spiritual harmonic. What sense, knowing, feeling, taste, or sensation is available in your harmonic that will disturb the malignant resonance? Which spiritual energetic forces when joined with this energy will blast the cancer in two? Use this knowledge and fire away!
4. With any intuitive method, if you are undergoing traditional treatments such as chemotherapy or radiation, or using herbs and supplements, attune to spiritual energetic forces that will accomplish one or both of these goals: (1) bolster the effectiveness of the process or material against the cancer and (2) support the healthy cells if they are exposed to toxicity. For instance, you can place an energy marker on the cancer cells and stick matching generative spiritual forces on the chemicals. Make both the same hue, so the chemicals will pursue only the cancer. After treatment, use degenerative forces on the chemicals to flush them from the body.

After using any of the above approaches, consult the "Working against the Cancer Cell" section under "Special Power Pathway Techniques" and use any of the exercises listed there.

Safeguarding Your Power

When introduced to the power pathway, some of my clients have felt too scared to use it. *What if I make a mistake?* they wonder.

What if I put the wrong force in the wrong place? There is another, related issue: because healing is a process rather than a one-time event, it might require only the temporary use of a particular spiritual energetic force — and when the need for that force is gone, you'll need to remove that force or else it could potentially create harm instead of benefit.

Here are a few methods for safeguarding yourself:

1. *Check your body.* Your body will tell you if you have misplaced a spiritual energetic force or pulled out one that is needed. You will feel uncomfortable, uneasy, or even ill. Know that you can always ask the Divine or your own higher self to correct the situation immediately, even if you don't understand exactly what is wrong.
2. *Use a time lock.* You can establish time parameters for any energetic work. For instance, let's say you insert a generative spiritual force in your immune cells. You don't want this force attached eternally to these cells — if it were, you could potentially create an autoimmune disease. When connecting the force, command that it remain linked until the objective is met, or set a certain time limit that seems right. Secure this time lock with a symbol, such as a cross with a circle.
3. *Align with your spiritual genetics.* Command that all spiritual energetic forces must attune to your spiritual genetics, or else they will simply detach or fall away.
4. *Utilize your etheric mirror.* Select only the spiritual energetic forces that attune to the template on your etheric mirror.
5. *Remember your personal harmonic.* Before placing or pulling a spiritual energetic force, you can check it against your personal harmonic. Also command that your energy system accept only forces that attune to this harmonic and for only as long as the relationship is beneficial.

Special Power Pathway Techniques

Here are a few techniques that make best use of the power pathway.

Setting the Seals

A more thorough description of this process is offered in *Advanced Chakra Healing: Energy Mapping*. Here are the six main steps:

Follow steps one and two in the "Five Steps for Safe Psychic Use" provided in the insert.

1. When you reach step three, "Conduct the goal," cleanse each chakra with breath or a golden-white light
2. Ask the Divine to send a guide to help you set your seals
3. Ask this guide to command each seal into its highest setting
4. Image a cross of equal arms either with or without a circle around it to lock the seal in place
5. Ask the guide to instruct you in using the seals

Cancer Healing with the Golden Kundalini The golden kundalini can help you access your serpent or red kundalini and bolster your basic life energy. Ask the Divine to start the process in love and faith. (For a complete description of how to initiate your golden kundalini, see *Advanced Chakra Healing*.)

Keying into Your Spiritual Harmonic Harmonics represent your major spiritual truth — for example, honesty, love, truth, or caring. You may have more than one key harmonic or spiritual attribute, but there is usually one main one. There are exercises for identifying your key personal harmonic in *Advanced Chakra Healing*; for a shortcut, think of the happiest moment in your life, then decide which spiritual truth best reflects the reason that you were so happy. Were you being honest? Truthful? Magical? The main truths that surface are related to your harmonic.

Reading the Book of Life for a Cancer-Free Life There are endless ways to journey through the Book of Life for healing. To call forth the book, simply command its presence, ask for a guide to assist you, or image the Book of Life that is your own and turn its pages to find your answers. Once you have it, you can do any of the following in addressing cancer.

Reading the Past Travel backward in time to find the reason you now have cancer, using the regression exercises in the insert or in *Advanced Chakra Healing*.

Reading the Present You can journey through the Book of Life to find the self who has the secrets to healing from cancer. Use the insert exercises on reading the present. Grasp the energy, knowledge, wisdom, cure, healing substance, or energy from this self and call forth a strong generative spiritual force to bring it into your body.

Reading the Future Is there a future self who is healed of cancer? Use the futuring exercise in the insert to travel through the Book of Life to find your future self and discuss the healing path. Bring this knowledge or healing energy back. Inspire it with spiritual energetic forces to follow the advice or effect the changes in your body.

If there isn't a healed future self, visit the self that died and ask if there are any alternatives or healing energies to be found in heaven. The worlds beyond life contain energies that we can tap into even in life. Ask an angel of death to assist in this process and transfer the healing or knowledge into the here and now.

Transmission through the Etheric Mirror Focus on the chakra (or seal, if set) that is closest to the cancer site. Call forth the generative spiritual force of connection, which will psychically look like a band of light. Connect the chakra or seal with the etheric mirror and command that the codes needed to heal the cancer transfer from that energy body into your physical body. Intensify this process using spiritual energetic forces that harmonize with your own spirit.

These codes can refresh and stabilize your tired healthy cells and immune system. They also compel existing DNA cells to either transform into healthy cells or die if they don't.

Working against the Cancer Cell As I've suggested, the power pathway is ideal for breaking up the resonance that is making cancer immutable. First use your intuitive faculties to hear, see, or sense the cancer cells. Begin by commanding forward a representative cancer cell, one of the master cells creating your condition. Command this cell to split into two halves, each resonating a different idea, energy, or structure. Now do one of the following:

- *Force with spiritual forces:* Attach two very different spiritual forces to each of the two cancer halves. Now set these spiritual forces against each other by establishing them in opposing spins, shapes, tones, colors, and speeds. Lock these forces into place so the cancer destroys itself.
- *Disempower with powers:* Raw powers can be used very effectively in opposition. As in working with forces, select two opposing powers, such as fire and water, and attach one to each of the two cancer halves. Now attach a generative spiritual force to one and a degenerative spiritual force to the other. One will draw the other out of the body.
- *Virtualize with virtues:* As with the other exercises, select two virtues that are different enough to seem opposing. Attach each to a half of the cancer and intensify their potency with spiritual forces or powers. The two "ideas" will battle and in doing so, cancel out the cancer.

I heartily recommend you try the above processes. I believe the future of medically based cancer healing will involve using similar processes, but with measurable energies, such as applying magnetics on one side of a tumor and electricity on the other.

Killing Your Cancer with Spiritual Genetics

As I stated earlier, your spiritual genetics have the correct programming to kill your cancer. Image yourself packing your spiritual genes into a tight ball and empowering this ball from the outside. First, pulse a spiritual force, virtue, or power that resonates with your harmonic inside of the ball. Second, spin an opposing spiritual energetic force outside of the ball. This opposition implodes and explodes the cancer at the same time. I predict that this basic idea will be used for another medically based cancer treatment at some time in the future.

Helpers on the Power Pathway

Now let's briefly meet a few of the beings and consciousnesses that stand by to assist you on the power pathway. (A more detailed description of these beings is available in *Advanced Chakra Healing*.)

Angels and teams of angels can work together toward a specific helpful objective, such as healing, cleanup, or restoration. They can help select the correct forces with which to work, show you pictures in the seals, and help you change forces. The angels of death can be very helpful in bringing back abilities that you "left on the other side" before you were born, or in summoning some of the energy from that other side.

Forms are entities that can transform energies from one form to another. The forms are also in attendance on the power, most typically the entities that are innately able to transform energy from one state to another. They can be used to change the form of your cancer into a nonmalignant mode. *With specific requests, a power player can also request the services of a form of being who has developed the skill of transformation. You might employ the services of a being capable of shifting a toxin to a benign element, for instance, to rid yourself from the long-term side effects.*

- *The Shining Ones* bring spiritual energies into the physical plane. For cancer, have them bring energies to sustain your healthy cells.

- *The Powers* send material energies into the spiritual dimensions. For cancer, have them convert cancer into the ethereal planes to make it disappear.
- *Archetypes* can help you hold your composure and strength while you battle cancer.
- *Muses* can generate your own spiritual harmonic, which you can use to hold the tones of the spiritual energetic forces you are using to erase the cancer or support your body, or to fixate the opposing energies used to break cancer's resonance.
- *The Ideals* assist in the correct placement and ordering of the virtues needed to support a healthy body.
- *The Virtues* command the properties of divine love, the greatest healing energy of all.
- *The Forces* stand ready to help you select, discard, or choose spiritual forces.
- *Masters and avatars* can help you make decisions and work clearly with the power pathway energies.

chapter eight

Energy Mapping on the Imagination Pathway

Where had I been that I didn't know about imaginary friends? I could see the point of it. How a lost part of yourself steps out and reminds you who you could be with a little work.

— Sue Monk Kidd, *The Secret Life of Bees*[1]

Travel the imagination pathway under these conditions:

- Your cancer is localized
- You are willing to accept responsibility for having and therefore changing the cancer
- In the past, you have made dreams come true with your imagination
- You believe that the past, present, and future all contain many possible paths
- You believe in the power of storytelling and pretending
- You have shamanic interests and abilities

- You seek to complement your work on another pathway with magical means
- You often use your sixth, eighth, or tenth chakra

The Imagination Pathway: The Mirror of Time

Have you ever watched a child play dress up? During the minutes spent pretending to be a doctor or Peter Pan or a mother, the child is convinced of the make-believe reality. Adults like to call this fantasy. Childcare experts insist that although these whimsies may not be harmful, they aren't "real."

Children disagree: "When I pretend, I *become* what I pretend to be!"

By the time we become adults, most of us have lost our belief in the magical. Science, interestingly, has reinvigorated the truth of the impossible, pointing out the existence of various dimensions and parallel universes, all possible because of quantum reality. If some quanta are only physical when seen, then where are they when we're not looking?

They are "there."

The impossible, the probable, the maybe, and the perhaps occupy their own universe, on the other side of the imagination mirror.

The world of possibilities has traditionally been the realm of the shaman. Shamans are the priest-healers, the medicine people, the soul healers, the supernatural mystics, of yesterday and today. Someone becomes a shaman through experiences that force an expansion of consciousness. Where the typical person might see light, the shaman also perceives shadows. Where the traditional medical doctor sees disease, the shaman might evaluate opportunity.

Shamans will instinctively understand quantum physics, for in the shamanic understanding, reality is an illusion. The world is full of invisible spirits and energies. Reality is simply a construct of what you believe it to be.

I recommend the imagination pathway for anyone who already identifies himself or herself as a shaman. If the mystical is new to you, I encourage you to attempt the imaginative anyway. Who knows what deep and hidden gifts linger in the "antiworld" of yourself that, if awakened, might provide the impetus or keys to healing?

Cancer and the Imagination Pathway

If cancer exists in your here-and-now body, then somewhere is a body that is cancer-free. Somewhere your healthy invisible self waits to be called forth, ready to exchange wholeness for disease.

The concept isn't as unbelievable as it sounds. Several studies of individuals with multiple personality disorder show that when a personality shifts, so sometimes do that person's bodily conditions. In one phase, a person might need and wear glasses, but his alter ego has twenty-twenty vision.

On the imagination pathway, cancer represents a condition that you have approved. You have consented to the idea of cancer, and so you are holding it in your body. Through this pathway, you can journey to a spacetime where you don't require cancer.

There are two main gatekeepers that you must pass, however, before you can make this flip: your subconscious and your spirit.

Gaining the support of both of these aspects of self is necessary to trade cancer for health through the "land of the looking glass" represented by the imagination pathway.

Tools and Healing on the Imagination Pathway

These are the concepts available on this pathway for healing cancer:

- Energies on the Imagination Pathway
- The Magic of Imagination
- Special Imagination Pathway Techniques
- Special Imagination Pathway Processes
- Helpers on the Imagination Pathway

Energies on the Imagination Pathway

There are no energy bodies on the imagination pathway. Playing in this realm basically involves remembering the basics of quantum physics. There are negative, positive, and neutral cancers and energies, and fast- and slow-moving energy. Analyzing down to this degree is helpful when playing in the looking glass.

Through each chakra, you have access to the imagination mirror. It has a sheen-like quality, and many people experience it as having three components:

1. A white side, upon which you see what is currently "true"
2. A black side, which draws from the "black hole" aspect of yourself and shows what could be possible (a black hole in space is impacted light that sucks energies into it)
3. An empty, neutral space in the middle from which you can make diagnoses and exchange energies between worlds

You use this mirror with your *imagination*—the part of your mind that can conjure images, pictures, and knowing. No matter which chakra you use to access the imagination mirror, your sixth and seventh chakras are almost always involved in the process. Your sixth chakra receives visions from all potential realities through its back side. The seventh chakra highlights your choices and, through the pineal gland, spins your selection into the universe. The imagination mirror within any chakra, however, is capable of exchanging energies from the antiworld to this world; from the realm of possibilities and stored potential to the world of the here and now.

Through the imagination mirror, you can accomplish the following:

- Identify what's going on here and now
- See into a different spacetime or antiworld to see what is possible
- Try on or test different life choices
- Neutralize a bad situation
- Exchange energies between the worlds
- Lock new changes into place

Two Useful Energy Tools

Two other energetic tools are especially useful on this pathway. One is an energy unit housed in the eighth chakra, which makes it a favorite for shamans seeking to investigate the cause of a problem. This is the Akashic Records, a collection of everything you've ever seen, done, or said; are experiencing now; or could experience based on future projections. Through these records you can visit the past to uncover causes for your cancer, try on various healing techniques available now to see if they will work, and connect with future time periods and selves to find new ideas.

The second energy tool helpful to the creative shaman is the second layer of the energy egg. This layer relates to the unconscious; it contains all the ideas and possibilities hidden there. The unconscious is more powerful than the conscious. If you can perceive new choices in the second layer and accept them, your unconscious can lock them in place.

The second layer of the energy egg can be visualized on the imagination mirror. You can also journey right into it and check out what possibilities lie in your own personal dreamland. Once you have selected one of the possibilities you find in this layer, connect it into the third layer of the energy egg and allow the Divine to bring it into your being.

Energy Symbology and Vibration

No matter which psychic technique you use on the imagination pathway, you are essentially working vibrationally. To control vibration, it is helpful to use energy symbols and techniques, so you don't make mistakes. In this way, you are upholding the potential of informed vibration.

In the imagination mirror, you can diagnose whether a cancer is essentially negative, positive, or neutral. As on the elemental pathway, negative cancers will be dark, have reverse spin, be held in boxy rather than circular shapes, and fit most of the other criteria spelled out in chapter 3. On the imagination pathway, however, you can notice where the reversing energy is going. Often it's being sucked into another energy world, though sometimes it's feeding another aspect of the self or someone else.

Positive cancers will be spinning forward and appear as they do on the elemental pathway, yet you'll have to watch carefully to see whether they are feeding a future self who isn't healthy and successful, a potentially harmful or unhealthy future, or someone else entirely.

Neutral cancers will look just plain stuck.

For all cancers, you can check for and work with the same concepts that you do on the elemental pathway: spin, coloration, symbology, tones, cords and other connections, and links to other planes, dimensions, zones, and more. The key is remembering that you can experiment before you lock a change into place. Even if you make a mistake, you can undo it!

I once worked with a California woman named Jackie who had just been diagnosed with uterine cancer. We played with the imagination mirror until she chose a different path than death. This was early in my exploration of these pathway concepts, so I didn't understand the need to lock healings into place. Her cancer disappeared, but returned two years later. During this time, I had briefly studied with a shaman from Siberia and was introduced to the idea of healing with symbols. Jackie and I performed the same maneuvers as we had years before and then secured the "healthy self" in a box. She went into remission and four years later is still in remission.

The Magic of Imagination

The imagination pathway can seem elusive and slippery, as the major instrument for action is absolutely invisible. Can you touch your imagination? Can you prove that your imagination is real? Even though we intuitively know that imagination exists, we don't understand the ways in which it magically transforms ideas into concrete reality.

Scientists suggest that anywhere from 80 to over 90 percent of the universe is composed of "dark matter." Dark matter is the invisible stuff that fills space. It is the energy of the void. It is also the substance used by the imagination to formulate reality.

Everything imaginable exists in potential, carried on waves or particles of possibilities. Many scientists believe that an "observer" must see or perceive a possibility as real before that possibility can manifest into practical reality. Your imagination is the imaging process involved in making a selection from the infinite and eternal realm of possibilities. It can program and sculpt dark matter, the energy of the void. This dark matter is then able to attract the energies that give it form and shape. In turn, the "observer" — which is the "you" behind the imagination — is affected by what you observe! Sometimes, by simply seeing a potential reality we can call it into being. Your "informed self" isn't fooled by the emptiness of dark matter. It knows that darkness is just a form of light, which means that light is the same as shaped darkness.

Want your imagination to work beneficially for you on this pathway? Follow these two steps:

1. Allow your imagination to show you what you really want from life
2. Learn how to use your imagination as a finely honed instru-

ment for directing energies, so you can get what you want out of life

Special Imagination Pathway Techniques

Here are a few of the techniques particular to the imagination pathway:

- *Locking in a Change.* You must lock imagination pathway changes into the imagination mirror, or else the energies transferred from one side of reality to another can slip back. Any symbol, shape, number, or tone will work, as will prayer or intention. If using a symbol or tone, you can select an energy lock that attunes to your personal harmonic or a basic lock such as a cross with equal arms within a circle.
- *Diagnosing from This Side of Reality.* Center yourself in the chakra involved in the cancer. Now look at the mirror in the center of the chakra and ask to see the cause of your cancer. You are peering into the mirror on this side of reality.
- *Healing from the Other Side of Reality.* Center yourself in the chakra involved in the cancer. Now flip into the antiworld of this chakra. Look at the antiworld mirror and acknowledge the energies or ideas allowing a cancer-free life. Gather and hold these energies as you pass back into this world. Now replace the cancer images in the this-world mirror with the cancer-free images you have brought from the antiworld. Send the cancer energies back into the antiworld. Lock in this change with symbols or intention.
- *Diagnosing through the Center of the Mirror.* There is an empty space in the center of the mirror. This is an ideal place to stand within when diagnosing through the imagination. Simply look through the mirror into this world to examine for the types and causes of cancer.
- *Healing through the Center of the Mirror.* After diagnosing from the center of the mirror, look through the mirror into the antiworld. What energies or alternative realities are avail-

able that could change your this-world reality of having cancer? Switch the energies from the antiworld with the cancer-causing energies of this world. Use energy locks, such as a symbol or strong intention, to hold this change in place.

- *Commanding Forces through the Center of the Mirror.* The center of an imagination mirror is a place of authority. Here, you can access the powers and forces of the power pathway to create masterful change. Simply command your desires from the center place and watch as the energies shift. Lock in your changes.

Special Imagination Pathway Processes

Here are a few processes and exercises that are helpful on the imagination pathway:

1. *Walking through the Mirror.* Bring your awareness into the primary cancer chakra and focus on the fact of having cancer. Gather up the energies causing cancer, then picture a large black door in the imagination mirror. Leap through this door with the cancer energy in hand. On this side of the mirror, you don't have cancer. Note the energy or idea that is responsible for this healthy state of affairs. Put this healthy energy into your heart and release the cancer energy into the antiworld. Now return to the here and now, noticing that your exit door is white. Shut the door firmly behind you and lock it, setting it with a symbol.
2. *Cipher Healing.* Center in your primary cancer chakra and ask to see within the this-world mirror the symbol or shape anchoring the cancer in this world. To better understand this symbol, work with the meanings in the chapter 5 insert or perform a regression or projection using the insert exercises. After comprehending the reasons for the cancer, decide if you are willing to learn a different way. If so, transfer the cancer energies into the antiworld and ask the Divine to translate healing energies into this world.

3. *Casing the Akashic.* Within the primary cancer chakra, look at the this-world mirror and ask for the unfolding of the Akashic Records. Now ask to review the situation that led to cancer. Now ask the Divine to completely flip the mirror, so you can see the antidote or cure for the cancer-causing situation. As you view the former situation in a new way, decide whether you are willing to accept the healed state. If you are, lock in the solution.
4. *Embracing the Shadow.* Within the primary cancer chakra, peer into the this-world mirror and ask to see the cancer. Now notice the shadowy energy around the cancer image. This is the Shadow Record of the cancer; it contains information about the hidden causes of the cancer. Examine the shadowy energy and command it to form images or provide information about the cancer. As you work with the unfolding data, look into the antiworld mirror for healing solutions; when you're ready, transfer these in. Lock in place when you are done.

Helpers on the Imagination Pathway

To gain assistance from the invisible on the imagination pathway, you must think of yourself as a shaman. Shamans can connect with any or all beings, as they can touch or visit any domain, whether currently real or not. The shamanic empire is a circus, with characters of all sizes, talents, and appearances. The shaman can actually work with any or all of the beings or energies described in the insert and in *Advanced Chakra Healing* — as can you, through the imagination.

Look to the hidden for beings that could be causing your cancer. For instance, a little water elemental might find your abdomen a substitute haven for its rightful home in a nearby lake. Some aspect of you might have felt sorry for the little creature and allowed it to move in. Here it is, bags and baggage and pets, including a pesky little amoeba that has thrown off your pH balance, so over time your colon cells mutated and now you have cancer. When contacting beings as helpers, remember to double-check all presenting sources for their potential helpful or harmful effects — just as shamans can be tricky, so can shamans be tricked!

A Note on Other Times

Sometimes cancer is the result of a need carried over from a past life. Believing in karma — the perceived need to justify mistakes by extracting payment from others or paying others back for our own errors — we may create a cancerous condition out of revenge or guilt. I once met a seventy-year-old man with lung cancer who in a past life had operated a coal mine. In that time period, he was responsible for the death of hundreds of men, women, and children from the toxic dust. He determined that he contracted his current cancer out of the seeming need to punish himself for hurting all these people. He had chosen a disease that mirrored that which had killed so many people once in his care.

Roger had brought an oxygen tank and an IV into my office with him. Despite the fact that his very advanced lung cancer had spread to his brain, he insisted that he was going to survive it. I didn't see how.

Upon hearing of the past-life involvement from his soul, he decided to forgive himself. I don't know whether Roger's miraculous recovery had to do with our session or his continual use of radiation treatment. I know only that even though he refused to quit his fifty-five-year smoking habit, his cancer went into complete remission. He died of emphysema three years later.

The imagination pathway is an ideal place to see exactly which parts of our soul might be writing a cancer script. Change the past; change the present; change how you see the past; create new opportunities for the future. Know that somewhere in the imagination lives a part of you that knows how to self-heal, another part that has healed, and yet another part that has never become ill. Take advantage of these magical realities, and move them into this one through the creativity of your mind.

chapter nine

Energy Mapping on the Divine Pathway

I slept and dreamed. I went into the church and Osia Theola's cave. Inside the cave my littlest brother and sister, Johnny and Rosy, were blowing bubbles, and the bubbles with their iridescent colors illuminated the darkness of the cave. Then I saw that each bubble was filled with stars, with galaxies, countless galaxies; each bubble was an island universe . . . universes glowing softly with the life of all creation.

— Madeleine L'Engle, *A House Like a Lotus*[1]

Travel the divine pathway under these conditions:

- The cancer is out of control
- You are in the very initial stages of a cancer
- Your need to accept unconditional love outweighs your fear of love
- You perceive that a higher reality exists and believe that you are only a breath away
- Your goal is unity, no matter what happens to the cancer
- You believe in the power of the Divine

- You desire to supplement work on another pathway through seeking spiritual truth
- You are willing to accept a miracle in any form in which it arrives
- You rely frequently on your third, seventh, or ninth chakra

The Divine Pathway: The State of Wholeness

The divine pathway is a state rather than a place. On the divine pathway, we come to realize that we are both fully human and fully divine, and that both are in fact the same state. We don't need to choose between our mundane, daily self and our enlightened, risen self. You already are one within yourself and therefore in unity with the world. This knowing leads to the state of *wakefulness.* Wakefulness is the heightened state of awareness that allows brokenness and wholeness to be seen as one and the same.

Terms used in spiritual circles for wakefulness include enlightenment, being born again, wisdom, mastery, *samadhi*, and consciousness, among others. The main difference between the Four Pathways concept of this advanced state and other ideas is that you don't have to follow a prescribed path or believe in any particular god or ideal to achieve the state. You have only to recognize your full capacity for humanity and divinity and to be willing to blend the two as one. This state is available through any of the pathways, but is easiest to associate and recognize on the divine pathway, as it is here that you deal mainly with spiritual concerns, rather than the specifics of your problems.

I call any work done on the divine pathway *illumination.* Illumination is the process of unfolding to wholeness. This is the process of healing on the divine pathway in general, regardless of the reason and the outcome. To illuminate does not require wakefulness, only the recognition that there is wholeness within the brokenness.

Cancer cells are broken cells. Underneath the brokenness is an unrevealed wholeness. Opening the brokenness to wholeness is the illumination — and therefore the healing — process.

Wakefulness involves taking another step. The wakeful attitude will recognize the brokenness as the key to wholeness. Cancer cells are broken, yet the fact of their existence is an invitation to new awareness and ultimate freedom. Therefore broken and whole are one and the same.

As I've said, you don't have to adopt this wakeful philosophy to heal physically on the divine, nor must you set wakefulness as a goal. You must merely illuminate or reveal the need for love and allow the power of love to heal you. Love is what makes us whole. This illumination process will change you, however, at a core level. Inevitably, divine pathway illumination leads to at least partial recognition of the wakeful state. Your recognition of truth might accompany a *Eureka!* moment or perhaps result from slower and more meditative awareness. Then again, you might discover that illumination and "waking up" are one and the same.

The prewakeful state is the image of living within a gold bubble. Here we function within time and space.

TO BE WAKEFUL IS TO BE AWARE. To be aware that not only is there unconditional love in the universe, but that the universe is established to meet our needs. When we're cold, there are blankets. When we're sad, there are smiles. When we're sick with cancer, there are ways to return all parts of us to harmony; and if we've never recognized harmony, we then assume an embrace into harmony.

The universe is established in a fail-safe form. Everything we need to heal or learn how to heal (in the here and now) is present in the Greater Reality. The Greater Reality includes the worlds beyond this one, the potential of other realities, and the history of the past.

The Greater Reality embraces the practical need for diet control and surgical maneuvers found on the elemental pathway, the supremacy of the supernatural assumed on the power pathway, the fantastical possibilities and mystical richness of the imagination pathway, and the assumption of divine blessing empowering the divine pathway. The wakefulness we allow on the divine pathway is a summation of the truths established on all the pathways — not only on this, the "most advanced" pathway.

Everything we've ever done or should have done or will or could do in our soul's entire eternal existence is occurring simultaneously. What I might have said a thousand years ago still lingers within this bubble, and affects what I could say a thousand years from now. This is my own personal Greater Reality. It is within the Greater Reality, although most of us believe that the Greater Reality is limited to our individual bubbles of existence.

We are each locked within our own golden galaxy. That is why we are inherently a lonely people. We don't know that everyone else is trying to cope with the same difficulties as we are. Within our own golden spheres, each of us must face the same basic seven challenges of humanity. These are symbolized in the bowls of existence described in the Christian New Testament Book of Revelation. It doesn't matter our age or gender, ethnic background or religion. We are all the same in that we must all deal with the difficulties of living dualistically, of thinking that everything has an opposite.

Within this circle, we travel the planes of existence along the chakras. We view various aspects of ourselves through these chakric lenses, seemingly reacting to some sort of external world but really still contained within ourselves. The auric field constitutes the boundaries between different types of experiences, feelings, and desires.

All the other pathways are contained within this single bubble, this sphere that surrounds each of us. The divine pathway is the only one that enables us to break out of the sphere while remaining inside of it. This is why the divine pathway is ideal for allowing the state of wakefulness, the recognition of wholeness within brokenness, of interconnectedness outside of the individual self, of illumination as the key to healing.

When we remain in the bubble and use what is within for healing, we are illuminating. We are our own "Greater Reality." When we accept that we are both inside and outside of the bubble, then we are moving into wakefulness. We are one with the Greater Reality.

If we're metaphorically enclosed within our golden fortification, we must become free in order to journey to or access the spiritual realms outside of the human dimension. One of the practical applications of these travels is to access powers for healing cancer. The chakras on the divine pathway are the key to the journey. You can journey the chakras and never leave the home of the earth plane or of your body.

Through the divine pathway, the chakras transform into twelve channels of light. These are like doorways of light passing through the gold walls surrounding us. Each of these channels of light is a truth available to us all. The ultimate truth, however, already lies deep within each of us. We merely need to awaken to it, to know that through these twelve basic truths we are linked to the entire universe, to nowhere and anywhere, and to everyone else. We are not isolated and alone within our seemingly safe spheres of gold. Upon this realization, we touch the hem of the garment of unity, the simplest and most profound of wakefulness truths. Even cancer cells are part of the greater unity, and can be enabled to reform to their original state.

Cancer and the Divine Pathway

Vibrationally, cancer doesn't match our basic harmonic.

Informationally, cancer doesn't line up with our spiritual intentions.

Because of these facts, cancer can actually serve as a way out of the narrow perspective that keeps us from being fully alive and vibrant. Because cancer doesn't play by the rules, it forces us to break the rules. *Lacking harmony and frequency, cancer can serve as a bizarre and magnificent invitation to freedom.* It pushes us to the edge of our desires, and there we must face our real need: to escape our golden prison to recognize unity.

Cancer can force us to insist upon freedom from the bubbles of consciousness containing us.

On the divine pathway, cancer will represent your chief issue, the one that keeps you locked into rigid beliefs that keep you from fully embracing divine love and acknowledging the divine love that completely encompasses you. The primary site of cancer points to the truth that will set you free — free to live in truth!

There are only a few steps in working the divine pathway, and of these, only two are really important:

1. See the challenge through the point of view of the cancer
2. Use the light of the pertinent chakra to heal into wholeness

Accomplishing these goals is the result of using the tools of the divine pathway toward healing.

Tools and Healing on the Divine Pathway

Of all the pathways, my favorite is the divine. When able to conceive the glory of wholeness and love, I have supported clients in achieving the most miraculous of healings. When people ask me how I was "able to heal them" when on this pathway, I can only reply, "I do absolutely nothing." That's not exactly true. You see, I trust the *system* of healing as much as the *process* of healing.

Here are the tools and concepts that allow you to use your own divinity in a systematic way:

- Energies on the Divine Pathway
- Petitioning on Purpose: The Key to Divine Healing
- Special Divine Pathway Healing Techniques
- Helpers on the Divine Pathway

Energies on the Divine Pathway

As on all pathways, there are energy bodies unique to the divine pathway. Those specific to this pathway are the *incandescent bodies*, including the *bodies of the eternal and the infinite*, which allow you to break free of the spacetime continuum; the *seven bowls of existence*, which hold humanity's greatest challenges (and, therefore, are our greatest teachers); the *seven channels of light*, which are the seven primary chakras, each representing a divine truth (to which I have added another five to assist with the top chakras); and the *twelve spiritual gates*, which are the evolved twelve auric fields.

These energy bodies are described in detail in *Advanced Chakra Healing: Energy Mapping*. The most important concept to grasp is how the bowls, channels of light, and twelve spiritual gates can help heal cancer, as can the energy egg introduced in the insert.

The Chakras and the Bowls

As on the other pathways, each type of cancer will relate to a specific chakra. Pinpointing the causative chakra helps you uncover the need underneath the problem. If you allow the light of this chakra to meet your need, you can potentially address the main issue of the cancer, which is reflected in the bowl relating to the primary chakra.

Look up your chakra that contains the primary cancer site, according to the information provided in chapter 4. Now track the need.

Chakra/Bowl: Channel of Light	*Need Shown by the Cancer*	*The Challenge Posed by the Cancer*
One	Self-definition, being "I"	Evil
Two	Being yourself	Death
Three	Self-determination	Judgment
Four	Connection through love	Power
Five	Communication through love	Suffering
Six	Evolution of self purpose	False miracles
Seven	Change through	Endings
Eight	Undoing what shouldn't have been	(See Gates)
Nine	Being hopeful	(See Gates)
Ten	Accepting what is now	(See Gates)
Eleven	Accepting grace	(See Gates)
Twelve	Truth of grace	(See Gates)

The Spiritual Gates The auric fields translate into the twelve spiritual gates on the divine pathway. These gates are extraordinarily important if you have cancer. The chakras can help you informationally, but the gates are necessary to restore law and order to cancer cells.

Remember that cancer cells have lost their ability to order themselves. Malignant cellular walls are loose and unstructured, and the genetic material is sloppy and inconsistent. Miraculous alterations of cancer involve the instant spiritual application of the boundaries and filtering capabilities of the auric fields on the divine pathway.

Each of the twelve spiritual gates relates to a specific chakra. Refer to *Advanced Chakra Healing* to learn how to incorporate the gates into your healing. Know that on the divine pathway, with the first seven chakras (channels of light) you will work both the chakra and its associated gate; beyond the seventh chakra, you will jump immediately to the auric field/gate.

The Energy Egg My favorite divine pathway tool is the third layer of the energy egg. This third layer links with the outer layer of the twelfth chakra and auric field, and so opens the door to the spiritual realms that lie outside of these bounds. Energies unknown to earth or even to this universe dwell in the spiritual realms, as well as energies that can be formed as needed. There are many ways to open the channels to these healing energies, which are actually spiritual waves, but the following is the easiest:

Acknowledge the presence of your spirit within you. From this center core, hold faith that the Divine completely surrounds you. Select the channel of light that relates most to your need and simply petition the Divine to open this channel between your center and the third layer of your energy egg. Because the third layer of the energy egg connects the spiritual realms to your physical body, these energies will flow through this channel and into your body.

Radiant Kundalini There is a special form of kundalini on the divine pathway: "radiant kundalini."

Within each and every cell, physical organ, and energy organ is a glowing, pulsing center. Most people psychically see this energy as a luminescent white. This white energy is the medium of spiritual truths; it could be described as the matter of spirit. Through this spiritual matter, divine truths accurate to your own destiny and path are transmitted from the Greater Reality. There is a special technique for using this kundalini for cancer healing in the upcoming section "Special Divine Pathway Healing Techniques."

Petitioning on Purpose: The Key to Divine Healing

To petition is to appeal to a higher authority or being. Petitioning is the secret to healing on the divine pathway.

Many people think that petitioning and praying are comparable. Petitioning is a form of prayer, but it's not exactly the same. Understanding this difference will help you make petitioning work for you.

To pray is to communicate to the Divine. Prayer involves any form of sharing or corresponding. It is a one-way effort, in that responses are returned through meditation. When petitioning, you are making a request. You are specifying exactly what you would like, and for what reasons. You don't need to meditate for a reply. Powerful petitioning assumes a supportive response.

Now, we would all like a universal power to respond to every one of our demands. Imagine how grand, if every one of our dreams would come true! Not only would I have a thousand pairs of shoes, but also closets to separate them by color. Petitioning on the divine pathway is a little more complicated than putting in an order in a restaurant and waiting to be served the requested meal. There are several factors involved, all of which fashion a spiritual petition that will obtain results. These can be reduced to understandings about the "who," "what," and "where" of petitioning.

The "Who" of Petitioning Everything and everyone are considered divine authorities on the divine pathway. The divine pathway recognizes the divinity and spiritual authority of all beings as equal in importance, though not necessarily equal in gifts and abilities. In the Greater Reality, all beings are joined through divine love. When you petition on the divine pathway, your plea is immediately transmitted throughout all dimensions of the Greater Reality. The beings that are able to respond to your needs most appropriately and in the most loving way will sense or feel your petition. Petition to the Divine, and the divinity within all other beings will respond.

The "What" of Petitioning All petitions are considered valid on the divine pathway. There is no heavenly review or comparative analysis to determine whose petitions are more vital or immediate. However, a petition will be transmitted according to truth; it will not necessarily "read" as you originally conceived it, which is why you might not always recognize that a response is related to the original petition.

The easiest way to think of the "what" of a petition is to peel away the layers of a request to its core. Deep in the core of a petition is a life pulse. Essentially, all petitions are a plea for love. This love-based energy carries the true message of the petition, and it is this truth that is conveyed through the grid lines of the Greater Reality, to be read or perceived by beings everywhere.

You might petition for a cancer healing and immediately undergo a healing crisis, such as a severe cold. This cold might be the answer to the petition, in that having the cold then forces you to meet a naturopath, who incidentally specializes in cancer!

The fact that petitions are psychically rewritten means that you can't make a mistake with a request. Nor can you err in to whom you direct a petition.

The "Where" of Petitioning Many religious people prefer to pray or petition in a place of worship. The intensity of shared belief is beneficial and can open our hearts for the prayer, meditation, and contemplation processes. There are no such requirements on the divine pathway, however, as everywhere is sacred ground, including your own body.

There is no place where God is not — even in a tumor site.

Special Divine Pathway Healing Techniques

Here are a few techniques for healing cancer on the divine pathway.

- *Opening the Channels of Light:* On the divine pathway, the first seven chakras convert into channels of light, while the top five transform in correspondence to certain spiritual gates. To bring about a conversion, you can center yourself in the place of the radiant kundalini within a chakra. Infuse your consciousness with this spiritual matter, then request that the Divine open the floodgates of this center to bring through all spiritual energies and truths needed to transform the chakra into an enlightened channel of light (or chakra linked with a spiritual gate). Perform this conversion for at least your primary cancer chakra, if not all chakras.

- *Channeling the Channels of Light:* Once you have transformed a chakra into a channel of light, you can direct the channeled energy for healing. Center in the radiating white light of your transformed chakra and think about the issue or problem affecting you. Acknowledge that this problem holds a nugget of opportunity, and that it is really a call for divine love. Now ask to embrace the energy needed to transmute the problem. Decide that you are willing to accept love in a way that doesn't involve cancer or another "negative" effect. Ask the Divine if there are any actions you need to take in daily life to lock such a change into reality, then follow any advice provided.
- *Lighting the Gates of Life:* Cancer cells lack solid cellular walls or genetic structure. The spiritual gates of light are available to establish correct form for any cell, organ, or physical process. To access a spiritual gate, center in the radiant core of your primary cancer chakra/channel of light. Now ask the Divine to connect you with the auric field linked with this chakra/channel of light. Ask the Divine if there is a learning required in order to convert this auric field into a spiritual gate, then pay heed to the advice. When you're done with this step, ask the Divine to transform your auric field into a spiritual gate. Now request that the Divine direct the energy of this gate into every bodily area that requires a structural change or strengthening. You can ask to watch as the Divine rearranges the biochemistry and energetics of the cancer cells, or any other areas that are being altered.
- *Radiation through Radiating:* On the elemental pathway, radiation is a valid way to kill cancer cells. Radiant kundalini

can potentially perform the same function, except that it kills the cancer with kindness, not poison. To direct the radiant kundalini for this purpose, center in the radiating spiritual matter in the primary cancer chakra/channel of light. Now ask the Divine to bring through the spiritual truths and energies needed to transform the cancer through the power of unconditional love. Feel this energy sweep through the center of the chakra/channel of light and beyond; acknowledge that you are receiving a full healing.

- *The Egg of Life:* The third layer of the energy egg is most partial to divine pathway work, as it links with spiritual energies that lie beyond the golden bubble that surrounds all interdimensional aspects of the self. From the center of your primary chakra/channel of light, ask the Divine to fully link you with the third layer of your energy egg. Now give permission for the Divine to open the windows of this egg into the Greater Reality beyond your golden bubble. The Divine will usher healing energies directly into your chakra/channel of light center. They will then ripple from this center through your radiant kundalini.
- *Cancer Makes a Request:* Cancer calls for a deeper form of love. For the duration of this exercise, you must suspend so-called logical thought and assume that the cancer cells are already in a whole state.

  Within this mind-set, center yourself in the primary cancer chakra/channel of light. Now ask for a representative cancer cell to appear in your mind's eye. Request that this cell show you its full beauty. Allow it to boast, to convey to you its truth. Ask the cell to specifically tell you how it is helping you achieve your spiritual destiny and goals. Now ask it if there is a different way that it (and its fellow cancer cells) can provide you with these gifts. As you negotiate with the cancer emissary, feel free to ask the Divine to serve as a nonpartisan mediator. When seeking a new contract, make sure that you ask what you must do to seal the deal. After completing the transaction, assure the cancer cell that you will keep your part of the bargain, as it will do the same for itself and the other cancer cells.

- *Divining on the Elemental Pathway*: This method is ideal for people who have single or multiple cancer sites and want to work on elemental issues through the divine perspective. It is best for working the emotional strongholds behind most negatively based cancers.

  To divine on the elemental pathway, know that the geographical site of the negatively based cancer contains feeling neuropeptides that are conjoined with harmful beliefs. To heal of cancers caused by emotional strongholds, you must separate the feelings (neuropeptides) from the harmful beliefs. Your feelings aren't the problem; your harmful beliefs are! Although you must discharge or change negative beliefs to allow healing from cancer, you must retain and essentially retrain your feelings to ensure such healing.

Feelings are guides. Feelings tell you what to do and how to respond to life's events. To fulfill this vital role, however, feelings must be blended with and fuel life-enhancing beliefs.

Therefore, to heal a cancer site from an emotional stronghold, you must free your captive feelings from their negative beliefs (thus releasing the stuck neuropeptides from their cancerous home), release or change these negative beliefs, and use the feelings for healing. To accomplish these goals, picture the cancer site in your body. Use your psychic vision to look at one of the receptor sites on a cell affected by the cancer. What feeling or set of feelings is locked into the receptor site? What harmful belief or beliefs are gluing these feelings to the cell? What life-enhancing beliefs need to replace any harmful beliefs, thus releasing the feeling neuropeptides?

Ask the Divine or your higher self to completely clear the energies of the negative beliefs from all aspects of yourself and to lock in the positive beliefs. Now ask the Divine or your higher self to gather the now-homeless feelings into a single ball of energy. Place this ball of energy in the radiating matter of the chakra/channel of light that corresponds to the cancer site. Your own spirit can now use these feelings for healing and healthy life responses as needed. It will actually select spiritual truths from the radiating chakra matter and link these truths with the feelings needed to spread the truths into your body, alerting the hypothalamus to which neuropeptides to produce.

Now ask the Divine or your higher self to gather energies from this chakra/channel of light center in order to repair the cancer site. You might want to image your higher self scooping these energies into a ball. then traveling to the cancer site, where it deposits the healing energies directly into the center of the cancerous tumor or organ. Ask the Divine to infuse this healing energy with the intensity of divine love and power needed to allow full healing.

Helpers on the Divine Pathway

The truth is that anything and everything in reality exist to assist you in healing through the divine pathway.

On this pathway, you could request help from the devil itself, but so long as you did so out of knowledge of the Divine and a genuine heart, only goodness would ensue. You can ask for angelic assistance and your neighbor might be prompted to assist. It doesn't really matter to whom you petition, for on this pathway everyone is unified.

There are special guides for this pathway, however. These include the angelic realms, as well as the following:

- *Aspects of the self* that are most helpful include your innocent child, who can heal the inner children; the God self, who can parent you; the future self, who is already healed; and the master self, who already has the tools to clear cancer
- *Masters and avatars* can share specific knowledge about your healing

- *Guardians* live outside of the golden bubbles occupied by our own interdimensional selves and assist with illumination
- *Religious figures* such as saints and ancestors can help you merge your divine and human selves

chapter ten

Healing through Wakefulness

Every true artist re-creates the art.

— Irving Stone, *The Agony and the Ecstasy*[1]

Healing beyond Death

When my father contracted lung cancer, surgery and radiation gave no benefit, and doctors predicted that he had six months to live.

When I was with him, he began to cry. I asked what he wanted me to pray for. He replied with one word, "Death."

"Cyndi, this is no life," he said. "I'm tired of moving between the bedroom and the dining room. It's time to go."

My father was dead within eight days, months earlier than his doctors predicted.

Why?

My father had decided that death would be a healing.

I attended his physical passing. It was one of the most holy and sacred experiences of my life. I felt the angels that attended. I psychically saw him slip from his body and greet his mother. I didn't witness my father's ending; I witnessed his birth into a new way of being. Since then, I have felt my father's invisible presence when I most needed help and comfort. He now provides me with love and encouragement far beyond that which I received when he was living.

Healing through the pathways isn't always going to result in bodily miracles. Devotion to self-healing, however, always leads to the pinnacle of the divine pathway — an invitation into wakefulness, a transcendence from dying and death to living and life.

The Reality of Death

We all linger under a death sentence. It is one thing to conceive of this fact and another to touch the reality of it. As stated by the main character in the book *Nectar in a Sieve*, "It is one thing to see a snake and another to touch it."[2]

Whether your cancer withdraws permanently or awaits to bite another day, whether your cancer goes into remission or progresses, whether you are miraculously cured or forced to face yet another poignant issue, cancer forces the truth of physical mortality. Who doesn't fear the inevitable end of this body, this time, these friendships, these goals and hopes and dreams?

What does the pathway philosophy have to say about "terminal" cancer?

The Mortality of the Here and Now and the Immortality of the Greater Reality

Cancer can't kill you. Our bodies die because they are done battling — and learning from — cancer, and it is time to live elsewhere. Death isn't only an ending; it is also a beginning.

We each have an immortal spirit. Your spirit resides simultaneously here, in your body, and beyond, in the "somewhere else" that is easiest to understand when dead. Unfortunately, most religions insist that you must die to get into the paradise, nirvana, or heaven that greets us beyond life. You are already within the Greater Reality. Heaven is here! You are *in* heaven, and heaven is within you! When you die, you simply interpret heaven in a different way.

To grasp this concept is easier for the mind than for the body. The body starts as dust and finally slips back into dust, while the rest of us whisks toward the stars. Yet the signs of our immortality are everywhere, and not just within the pages of sacred documents or within the words of spiritual prayers or from the mouths of pastors delivering hopeful sermons.

> *The most important sign of eternity and immortality is your ability to love. You can love while alive, and you will love after you have finished passing through this place called life.*

The Four Pathways philosophy says that we must look not *to* our death but *through* death to the real nature of life: wakefulness.

The Wakeful State of Illumination

To live in the state of wakefulness is to accept that you will surely die sometime. To be wakeful is to know that death isn't an end, only a new beginning.

To be wakeful is to move through cancer as if you don't have it, knowing that it is providing you immeasurable favors today. To be wakeful is to know the universe as good, even to the end degree of accepting some goodness in cancer. In the end, to be wakeful is to be yourself, knowing that no matter your state of health or ill health, you simply "are." To be wakeful is to be more than your cancer, even as you see the cancer as more than itself. Be awake on this journey of self-healing, and all the universe will bend to help.

As the poet Rumi once said, and the Divine always says, "I make medicine out of your pain."[3]

Conclusion: The Chakras and Immortality

I am a great believer in chakra-based healing. There must be some reason that so many cultures over thousands of years have perceived and taught about these wheels of power. Yet chakras are only tools, elevators to take us through the appearance of the physical into a greater beyond.

As you progress up the pathway system, the chakras themselves evolve and change in nature, vibration, and function. On the elemental pathway, they are solid and spinning vortexes that mix chemicals, nutrients, minerals, gases, and elements with the ethers of spirit and dreams. I remember a vision I had one night, in which I saw for the briefest of moments the true composition of the chakras from an elemental point of view. They really were made of physical bits of matter, as well as the cloudy material of the heavens.

The same quanta occupying the elemental universe pulse within the realm called the power pathway. The same quanta — these bytes of matter that are the submatter of creation — exist within us.

On the power pathway, chakras evolve into seals — lenses that catch the stardust of forces that you can focus for personal gain.

Releasing the ideas of what is natural and even what is supernatural, we transcend through the chakras into the imagination. Imagination refers to the ability to form ideas and images in the mind, especially regarding things never before seen or thought of. Consider the first chapters of the Christian, Judaic, and Islamic scriptures. Here we read the story, or at least a storytelling, of how the physical world came to be:

Within each of us is the necessity to respond to the death call of cancer by singing about our lives.

"God, at the beginning of time, created heaven and earth. Earth was still an empty space, and darkness hung over the deep . . . Then God said, let there be light . . . And God said, Let us make man, wearing our own image and likeness . . . Man and woman both, God created them."

God created. We are made in the image of God; therefore, we create. Within each of us lies the pathway of imagination, for as we are beings that were once imagined and now exist, so are our imaginations the means to create and recreate our existence.

Within us all is the ability to search the darkness of despair, not only to find a light, but also to create one.

On the imagination pathway, the chakras become mirrors — not to massage and mutate reality, but to forge the attitudes that make us true artists of reality.

As the chakras evolve, we resolve our issues through them. Channels of light, they enlighten the deepest pains imaginable, the so-called bowls that hold the bitterest of potions. We all drink from these cups of evil and death, power and pain. No one is spared. Whether we face human reality through the truth of cancer or heart disease, loss of a loved one, or boredom, we all suffer from the same drink. The secret is one that the spiritual leaders of the world will never tell you: these bowls, the symbols of our pain and agony, are each a holy grail.

Pain makes us suffer; it seldom brings pleasure. In the drinking of pain, you don't learn the opposite of pain; rather, you learn how to create from pain.

If you are dying, you don't necessarily receive more time (although you might). The only guarantee is that through accepting the life within us, we are provided the opportunity to shape our lives into something monumental. Into something true. Into art.

The universe presents us with all the challenges needed to face our human indignities and to claim our divinity. The holy grail — the so-called cup that holds the liquid of immortality — has already been offered you, through the very existence of the chakras and the truths they allow you to face. As a channel of light, claim your right to be that light and to create from that light through the rest of your life — and beyond.

As author Joanne Harris suggests, simply "Travel far enough . . . and all rules are suspended."[1]

Pathway Reading Lists

Part I

Achtenberg, Jeanne, *Imagery in Healing*, Boston: Shambhala Publications, Inc., 1985.

Aczel, Amir, *Entanglement*, New York: The Penguin Group, 2003.

Austin, James, M.D., *Zen and the Brain*, Cambridge, MA: The MIT Press, 1999.

Benson, Herbert, M.D., *Timeless Healing, New* York: Scribner, 1997.

Braden, Gregg, *The God Code*, Carlsbad, CA: Hay House, 2004.

Buckman, Robert, Dr., *What You Really Need to Know about Cancer*, Baltimore, MD: The Johns Hopkins University Press, 1997.

Challem, Jack, *The Inflammation Syndrome*, Hoboken, NJ: John Wiley & Sons, 2003.

Chopra, Deepak, M.D., *Creating Health*, New York: Houghton Mifflin, 1995.

Couden, W. Lee, M.D., Diamond, John, M.D., with Goldberg, Burton, *Definitive Guide to Cancer*, Tiburon, CA: Future Medicine Pub., Inc., 1997.

Dale, Cyndi, *New Chakra Healing*, St. Paul, MN: Llewellyn Publications, 1998.

Dollingner, Malin, M.D., Mulvihill, Sean J., M.D., Rosenbaum, Ernest H., M.D., and Tempero, Margaret, M.D., *Everyone's Guide to Cancer Therapy: How Cancer Is Diagnosed, Treated, and Managed Day-to-Day*, 4th Ed., Kansas City: Andrews McMeel Pub., 2002.

Dossey, Larry, M.D., *Reinventing Medicine*, San Francisco: HarperSanFrancisco: 1999.

Eyre, Harmon J., M.D., Lange, Dianne Partie, and Morris, Lois B., *Informed Decisions: The Complete Book of Cancer Diagnosis, Treatment, and Recovery*, New York: American Cancer Society, 2002.

Gerber, Richard, M.D., *Vibrational Medicine*, Rochester, VT: Bear & Company, 2001.

Greene, Brian, *The Fabric of the Cosmos*, New York: Vintage Books, 2004.

Halpern, Paul, *The Great Beyond*, Hoboken, NJ: Wiley, 2004.

Hubbard, Barbara Marx, *Conscious Evolution*, Novato, CA: New World Library, 1998.
Hunt, Valerie, *Infinite Mind*, Malibu, CA: Malibu Publishing, 1996.
Liungman, Carl, *Dictionary of Symbols*, Santa Barbara, CA: ABC-Clio, Inc., 1991.
Mario, Livio, *The Golden Ratio*, New York: Broadway Books, 2002.
McCartney, Francesca, Ph.D., *Body of Health: The New Science of Intuition Medicine for Energy and Balance*, Novato, CA: Nataraj Publishing, 2005.
Orloff, Judith, M.D., *Second Sight*, New York: Warner Books, 1997.
Oschman, James L., *Energy Medicine*, Philadelphia, PA: Churchill Livingstone, 2000.
Pearsall, Paul, M.D., *The Heart's Code*, New York: Broadway, 1999.
Ross, Julia, M.A., *The Diet Cure*, New York: Penguin Books, 1999.
Russell, Peter, *From Science to God*, Novato, CA: New World Library, 2003.
Siegel, Bernie S., *Love, Medicine and Miracles*, New York: Harper & Row, Publishers, Inc., 1986.
Steiner, Rudolf, *An Outline of Occult Science*, Hudson, NY: The Anthroposophic Press, 1972.
Talbot, Michael, *The Holographic Universe*, New York: HarperCollins Publishers, 1991.
Webb, Stephen, *Out of This World*, New York: Praxis Publishing Ltd., 2004.
Weil, Andrew, M.D., *Health and Healing*, New York: Houghton Mifflin Co., 1998.
Wolf, Fred Alan, Ph.D., *Taking the Quantum Leap*, New York: Harper & Row Publishers, 1981.
Zukav, Gary, *The Seat of the Soul*, New York: Simon & Schuster, 1989.

Additional Resources

What the Bleep Do We Know? Twentieth Century Fox, 2004, now on video-DVD.

Part II

Elemental

Amen, Daniel, M.D., *Change Your Brain, Change Your Life*, New York: Three Rivers Press, 1998.
Balch, James F., M.D., and Stengler, Mark, N.D., *Prescription for Natural Cures*, New York: John Wiley & Sons, 2004.
Ballentine, Rudolph, M.D., *Radical Healing*, New York: Three Rivers Press, 1999.
Bradshaw, John, *Bradshaw On: The Family*, Deerfield Beach, FL: Health Communications, Inc., 1988.
Brand-Miller, Jennie, Ph.D., Colagiuri, Stephen, M.D., Foster-Powell, Kaye, M., and Wolever, Thomas M.S., M.D., Ph.D., *The New Glucose Revolution*, New York: Marlowe & Co., 2003.

Brennan, Barbara Ann, *Hands of Light*, New York: Bantam, 1988.
Gerber, Richard, M.D., *A Practical Guide to Vibrational Medicine*, New York: Perennial Currents, 2001.
Hay, Louise, *You Can Heal Your Life*, Carlsbad, CA: Hay House, 1999.
Jacka, Judy, N.D., *The Vivaxix Connection*, Charlottesville, VA: Hampton Roads Publishing Company, 2000.
Johnson, Steven, *Mind Wide Open: Your Brain and the Neuroscience of Everyday Life*, New York: Scribner, 2004.
Kabat-Zinn, Jon, Ph.D., *Full Catastrophe Living*, New York: Delta Trade Paperbacks, 1990.
Kushi, Michio, *The Cancer Prevention Diet*, New York: St. Martin's Griffin, 1993.
Lowry, Lois, *The Giver*, New York: Laurel-Leaf Books, 1993.
McCabe, Vinton, *Practical Homeopathy*, New York: St. Martin's Griffin, 2000.
Morra, Marion, and Potts, Eve, *Choices: The Most Complete Sourcebook for Cancer Information*, New York: Quill, an imprint of HarperCollins Pub., 2003.
Murray, Michael N.D., and Pizzorno, Joseph, N.D., *Encyclopedia of Natural Medicine*, New York: Three Rivers Press, 1998.
Null, Gary, Ph.D., *The Clinician's Handbook of Natural Healing*, New York: Kensington Books, 1997.
Pert, Candace, Ph.D., *Molecules of Emotion*, New York: Scribner, 1999.
Seuss, Dr., *My Many Colored Days*, New York: Alfred Knopf, book design 1996.
Sheldrake, Rupert, *A New Science of Life*, Rochester, VT: Park Street Press, 1995.
Varona, Verne, *Nature's Cancer-Fighting Foods*, New York: Reward Books, Penguin Putnam Inc., 2001.

Power

Bauval, R., and Hancock, G., *Keeper of Genesis*, London: Heinemann, 1996.
Berg, Yehuda, *The Power of Kabbalah*, Los Angeles, CA: Kabbalah Centre Intl., 2004.
Berrisford-Ellis, Peter, *The Druids*, London: Constable, 1994.
Campbell, Joseph, and Moyers, Bill, *The Power of Myth*, New York: Doubleday, 1988.
Cannon, Dolores, *Jesus and the Essenes*, Bath: Gateway Books, 1992.
Castaneda, Carlos, *Tales of Power*, New York: Simon & Schuster, 1974.
Cawthorne, Thomas, and Franke, Sylvia, *The Tree of Life and the Holy Grail*, London: Temple Lodge, 1996.
Cooper, Susan, *The Dark Is Rising*, New York: Aladdin Paperbacks, 1973. (As well as the rest of The Dark Is Rising series.)
Doresse, J., *The Secret Books of the Egyptian Gnostics*, Paris: Librarie Plon, 1958.
Emoto, Masaru, *The True Power of Water*, Hillsboro, OR: Beyond Words, 2005.
Fortune, Dion, *Esoteric Orders and Their Work*, Wellingbro, UK: Aquarian Press, 1987.

Fox, Matthew, *The Original Blessing*, Sante Fe, NM: Bear & Co., 1983.
Gardner, Laurence, *Genesis of the Grail Kings*, Gloucester, MA: Fair Winds Press, 2002.
Hawkins, David, *Power versus Force: The Hidden Determinants of Human Behavior*, Carlsbad, CA: Hay House, 2002.
Heselton, Philip, *The Elements of Earth Mysteries*, Shaftesbury: Element Books, 1991.
Hunbatz, Men, *The Secrets of Mayan Science/Religion*, Santa Fe, NM: Bear & Company, 1990.
Mails, Thomas, *Fools Crows Wisdom & Power*, Tulsa, OK: Council Oaks Books, 1991.
Morgan, Marlo, *Mutant Message Down Under*, Lees Summit, MO: MM Co., 1991.
Myss, Carolyn, Ph.D., *Invisible Acts of Power: Personal Choices That Create Miracles*, New York: Free Press, 2004.
Pullman, Philip, *The Golden Compass*, New York: A Yearling Book, Dell Yearling, 1995.
Rowling, J.K., *Harry Potter and the Sorcerer's Stone*, New York: Scholastic Inc., 1997.
Shah, Idries, *The Way of the Sufi*, London: Penguin, 1982.
Tolle, Eckhart, *The Power of Now*, Novato, CA, and Vancouver, BC, CAN: New World Library and Namaste Publishing, 1999.
Trungpa, Choygam, *The Sacred Path of the Warrior*, Boston: Shambhala, 1984.
Webster, Richard, *Spirit Guides and Angel Guardians*, St. Paul, MN: Llewellyn Publications, 1998.

Imagination

Allende, Isabel, *Kingdom of the Golden Dragon*, New York: HarperCollins Publishers, 2004.
Attanasio, A.A., *The Serpent and the Grail*, New York: Harper Prism, 1999.
Atwater, P.M.H., *Future Memory*, Charlottesville, VA: Hampton Roads, 1999.
Castaneda, Carlos, *The Art of Dreaming*, New York: Harper Collins Publisher, 1993.
Dahl, Roald, *Charlie and the Chocolate Factory*, New York: Puffin Books, 1964.
Eliade, Mircea, *Shamanism: Archaic Techniques of Ecstasy*, Princeton, NJ: Bollingen Foundation, 1964.
Harman, Willis, Ph.D., and Rheingold, Howard, *Higher Creativity*, New York: The Putnam Publishing Group, 1984.
Johnson, Crockett, *Harold and the Purple Crayon*, New York: HarperCollins, 1955.
Kaku, Michio, Ph.D., *Hyperspace: A Scientific Odyssey through Parallel Universes*, New York: Anchor, 1995.
Katz, Richard, *Boiling Energy*, Cambridge, MA: Harvard College, 1982.
Newton, Michael, Ph.D., *Journey of Souls*, St. Paul, MN: Llewellyn Publications, 1994.
Perkins, John, *The World as You Dream It*, Rochester, VT: Destiny Books, 1994.
Popescu, Petru, *Amazon Beaming*, New York: Penguin Books, 1991.

Skully, Nicki, *The Golden Cauldron: Shamanic Journeys on the Path of Wisdom & Power*, Rochester, VT: Bear & Company, 1991.
Some, Malidoma Patrice, *Of Water and the Spirit*, New York: The Penguin Group, 1994.
Villoldo, Alberto, Ph.D., *Shaman, Healer, Sage*, New York: Harmony, 2000.
Zukav, Gary, *The Dancing Wu Li Masters*, New York: Bantam Books, 1979.

Divine

Bly, Robert, ed., *The Soul Is Here for Its Own Joy*, New York: HarperCollins, 1995.
Brinkley, Dannion, *The Secrets of the Light*, Henderson, NV: HeartLIght Productions, 2004.
Childre, Doc, and Martin, Howard, *The HeartMath Solution*, San Francisco: HarperSanFrancisco, 2000.
Chodron, Pema, *When Things Fall Apart*, Boston: Shambhala Publishers, 2002.
Cleary, Thomas, *The Taoist I Ching*, Boston: Shambhala Publishers; 2002.
Coelho, Paulo, *The Alchemist*, San Francisco: HarperSanFrancisco, 1994.
De Sainte Exupery, Antoine, *The Little Prince*, New York: Harcourt, Inc., 1943.
Douglas-Klotz, Neil, *Prayers of the Cosmos*, San Francisco: HarperSanFrancisco, 1990.
Frankl, Viktor, E., M.D., *The Doctor and the Soul*, New York: Vintage Books, 1973 ed.
Gallico, Paul, *The Snow Goose*, New York: Alfred A. Knopf, 2000.
Hanh, Thich Nhat, *Living Buddha, Living Christ*, New York: Riverhead Books, 1995.
Hughes, Gerard, *God of Surprises*, Boston: Cowley Publishers, 1993.
Johnson, George, *Fire in the Mind: Science, Faith, and the Search for Order*, New York: Vintage Books, 1995.
Kelsey, Morton, *Healing & Christianity*, Minneapolis, MN: Augsburg Press, 1995.
L'Engle, Madeleine, *A Wrinkle in Time*, New York: Yearling Books, Random House Children's Books, 1962.
Lewis, C.S., *The Lion, The Witch and the Wardrobe*, New York: Harper Trophy, 1950. (As well as the Chronicles of Narnia series.)
Shealy, C. Norman, M.D., *Sacred Healing: The Curing Power of Energy & Spirituality*, Lanham, MD: Element Books Ltd., 1999.
Templeton, John M., and Herrmann, Robert, *The God Who Would Be Known: Revelations of the Divine in Contemporary Science*, Radnor, PA: Templeton Foundation Press, 1999.
Walsch, Neale Donald, *Tomorrow's God: Our Greatest Spiritual Challenge*, New York: Atria, 2004.
Wiesel, Elie, *Wise Men and Their Tales*, New York: Schocken Books, 2003.

Additional Resources

Brain Sync audio programs and CDs. Spirituality series. www.brainsync.com.

Endnotes

Chapter 1

1. Dan Brown, *Angels and Demons* (London: Corgi Books, 2000), 126.
2. Paul Pearsall, Ph.D., *The Heart's Code* (New York: Broadway Books, 1988), 13.
3. Kurt Vonnegut, *Kurt Vonnegut: The Collected Works* (New York: William Heinemann Inc. and Octopus Books, published through Delacorte Press/Seymour Lawrence, 1980), 569.
4. Amir Aczel, *The Mystery of the Aleph* (New York: Pocket Books, 2000), 37.

Chapter 2

1. Dean Koontz, *By the Light of the Moon* (New York: Bantam Books, 2002), 284–85.
2. Clifton Leaf, "The War Against Cancer," *Fortune Magazine* 22 (March 22, 2004): 78.
3. J.C. Bailar III and E. M. Smith, "Progress Against Cancer?" *New England Journal of Medicine* 314, (1986): 1226–32.
4. Curt Suplee, "The Speed of Light is Exceeded in Lab: Scientists Accelerate a Pulse of Light," *The Washington Post* (July 20, 2000).
5. Vertergaard Lene Hau, "Frozen Light," *Scientific American* (May 2003): 44–51.
6. Lee Smolin, "Atoms of Space and Time," *Scientific American* (January 2004): 73.
7. James. L. Oschman, *Energy Medicine* (New York: Churchill Livingstone 2000), 18.
8. Richard Gerber, M.D., *A Practical Guide to Vibrational Medicine* (New York: HarperCollins, 2000), 227.
9. Oschman, *Energy Medicine*, 143–144.
10. Gerber, *A Practical Guide to Vibrational Medicine*, 289.

Chapter 3

1. Andrew Clements, *Things Not Seen* (New York: Puffin Books, 2002), 249.
2. W. Wayt Gibbs, "Untangling the Roots of Cancer," *Scientific American*, Special Edition, Volume 14, Number 3 (2004): 69.
3. Houppert, Karen, "Go Ahead, Get Angry," *Organic Style*, (April 2005): 92.
4. Talbot, Michael, *The Holographic Universe* (HarperCollins Publishers, 1991), 213–16.
5. Doc Lew Childre, *Freeze Frame* (Boulder Creek, CA: Planetary Publications, 1994), 42–49.
6. James L. Oschman, *Energy Medicine* (New York: Churchill Livingstone, 2000), 49.
7. Phillip Day, *Cancer* (Kent, U.K.: Credence Publications, 2003), 30–46.
8. Leaf, Clifton, "The War against Cancer," *Fortune Magazine*, 22 (March 22, 2004): 78.

9. Michael Lerner, *Choices in Healing* (Cambridge, MA: MIT Press, 1996), 93.

Chapter 4

1. Dean Koontz, *By the Light of the Moon* (New York: Bantam Books, 2002), 284–285.
2. Rosalyn Bruyere, "Hunt's Case Studies," in *Wheels of Light*, (Sierra Madre, CA: Bon Productions, 1989), 247–259.
3. Richard Gerber, M.D., *Vibrational Medicine*, (Santa Fe: Bear & Company, 1988), 111

Chapter 5

1. Susan Cooper, *The Dark Is Rising* (New York: Aladdin Paperbacks, 1973), 11.

Chapter 6

1. Joanne Harris, *Blackberry Wine* (London: Transworld Publishers, 2000), 206.

Chapter 7

1. Joanna Pitman, *On Blondes* (New York: Bloomsbury, 2003), 4.

Chapter 8

1. Sue Monk Kidd, *The Secret Life of Bees* (New York: Penguin Books, 2003), 246.

Chapter 9

1. Madeleine L'Engle, *A House Like a Lotus* (New York: Dell Publishing, 1984), 306.

Chapter 10

1. Irving Stone, *The Agony and the Ecstasy* (New York: Signet Books, 1961), 437.
2. Kamala Markandaya, *Nectar in a Sieve* (New York: Penguin Group, 2002), 14.
3. Coleman Barks, *The Essential Rumi* (San Francisco: HarperSanFrancisco, 2004), 310.

Conclusion

1. Joanne Harris, *Blackberry Wine* (London: Transworld Publishers, 2000), 87.

Index